Medical Rape

State Authorised German Perversion

I0118142

Lars G Petersson

chipmunkapublishing

the mental health publisher

Lars G Petersson

All rights reserved, no part of this publication may be reproduced by any means, electronic, mechanical photocopying, documentary, film or in any other format without prior written permission of the publisher.

Published by

Chipmunkapublishing

PO Box 6872

Brentwood

Essex CM13 1ZT

United Kingdom

http://www.chipmunkapublishing.com

Copyright © Lars G Petersson 2010

Chipmunkapublishing gratefully acknowledge the support of Arts Council England.

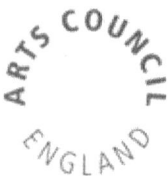

Medical Rape

Acknowledgement

This book has been written for all the men who have suffered as a result of abusive medical examinations by military institutions and their civilian associates. It has been written in the hope that young people today shall not one day have to join the ranks of older sufferers. Without the unwavering support of my wife Josephine and the help of members of the BASTA campaign (campaign against military abuse) it would never have been possible for me to finish this work. Thanks to all of you.

Lars G Petersson, London July 2010

Lars G Petersson

Medical Rape

Better Check it all Works

She has got nothing on but a pair of knickers. The same goes for the other few young women in the waiting room. They are all so lightly dressed - and they all seem uncomfortable with the situation. Constantly men with files are running back and forth, and some of them can't help having a quick glance at the young ladies while passing.

After a long waiting at last it is Ursula Müller's turn. A man in a white coat stands in the door and calls her name. For the young woman it's indeed quite stressful to walk across the room in such an almost naked state. However, she's got no choice: after all, the examination for which she has come is a legal duty, and if she hadn't turned up she could not only have been punished but, worse, police would have 'escorted' her to another 'appointment'. Would the young woman have tried to avoid even that, she could very well have ended up in prison. Not a nice prospect really. No, going to jail Ursula wouldn't fancy. After all, she hasn't done anything bad. In fact she has done nothing at all. She has only grown into an adult or at least almost so - that's all. Seventeen she is, and in another few months she will be eighteen.

As the young woman then finally enters the examination room she finds herself in the company of two men: one whom she believes is a doctor and another she reckons must be his assistant. However, it's all a guess; none of them has intro- duced themselves.

Now something will happen that Ursula never will forget: her body will be thoroughly inspected and assessed - that's why she was 'asked' to come. Nothing will go undetected: head to toe it will be - mouth, teeth, breasts... just everything. In the middle of it all, half naked as she is, she will be asked to do twenty squats - with blood pressure before and after. Bit strange really - as if her blood pressure, due to the forced condition, hasn't gone through the roof already, regardless of being 'asked' to do squats or run a marathon.

After the young woman had been through all the initial proce- dures something comes that she has feared all along, actually for years. The last protection of her privacy will be removed. 'Take off your knickers, please!' Ursula's cheeks turn red and hot; she stands there helpless, doesn't know what to do. No, she doesn't want to do that. 'I don't want to be stark naked in front of two men,' she thinks to herself. It's too embarrassing a prospect. 'No, don't do it!' a subconscious voice screams at her.

Ursula is gripped by a terrible anxiety as she notices the young man behind the desk looking in her direction with a slight smile on his face. In the same moment the now impatient doctor repeats his order. With sharpness in his voice he commands: 'KNICKERS OFF!' The young girl at this point obviously see no option but to do as she is told. The little resistance she might have had is gone; she is defence-less. Now she is completely naked; she stands in the middle of the room, totally exposed; she feels the last slight protection of her human dignity has disappeared. She wishes she could sink through the floor; she feels so embarrassed and humiliated.

Ursula's most intimate parts of the body are now to be zealously scrutinised und inspected. The doctor starts to check her genitals, and he is doing it with great thoroughness. After all, it must be tested as to its functionality, or so it seems. He repeats his movements not just once but twice. In this moment Ursula's most private parts sort of belong to another person, something she would never have allowed had she had had a choice. Then another order is heard: 'turn around, bend forward and spread the buttocks!' Automatically, now without resistance, the girl does as she is told. Her bum is now being thoroughly inspected with a little torch. She is, however, lucky: a finger in her anus she is spared (other 'patients' have to experience that to).

Ursula has had more luck this day as she has only been inspected by one doctor not two, which often can be the case. Sometimes also two assistants can be present, as new staff from time to time have to be trained for the job. Indeed, it can be quite crowded around the 'object'.

Finally Ursula is allowed to put back on her knickers and leave the room. As she returns to the waiting area the other girls out there note that her face is like a tomato. Rest assured, they will soon, one after another, have the same experience.

Medical Rape

Of course this story never happened as it was here told. After all, that's not a way to treat young women. Completely out of order it would have been - impossible, simply perverse. Most people would share that view. Some might even ask: what fucking pervert has written such nonsense?

Yes, what do I actually want to tell with such a story? In fact this: that a story like the one about Ursula not exclusively is to be found in the sick fantasy world of a sadomasochistic old bugger - actually it has all a very real background. To make the story true we only need to swap the genders of all people involved. Having done so, it all turns into reality. Then we can also give it a name: a 'military medical induction' or, in German, '*musterung*'. We now talk about a legally enforced medical where young men, mainly by women, as cattle on a market place, are examined, inspected and assessed for forced military or civilian service.

At least one thousand times this scenario is repeated all across Germany every day all year around. The number of similar examinations and controls are, however, much higher, as not only will young men be selected this way or discarded as possible candidates for forced service, a process which can mean repeated requests to make one self available for scrutiny, but in all barracks and by all civilian authorities responsible for 'employing' conscientious objectors all of it in every detail will be repeated not only when starting but also when leaving service - and sometimes even in between. On top of that comes thousands of identical checks of young men who, for one reason or another, totally voluntarily or due to civilian unemployment, has chosen the military as a temporary or permanent employer. Also these individuals (contrary to their female colleagues...) are constantly exposed to the same kind of intrusive 'examinations'.

Of course, testicles and backsides of young people can hardly have anything to do with defence of a country. Even for the defence authorities themselves that seems to make sense, as, certainly, nothing in this area would serve as a reason for anybody to be excluded from forced service or for that sake not to be accepted as a volunteer. Despite that, however, eager officials continue to order these parts of the body to be checked as to their optimal function - as said not only repeatedly before but also after ending the service. After all, the foreskin might have got stuck since the last examination.... Better make sure it hasn't.

No matter what, how odd it all might seem, all what we talk about here is in Germany fully legitimate and established. Again and again the call sounds: strip! Again and again the state and its willing helpers reach out after young men's testicles and foreskins, and again and again they are commanded to turn around, bend forward and spread their buttocks. And (isn't it remarkable?), all of a sudden nobody seems to see a problem in it any longer. Nobody looks at it as an assault - as they certainly would had 'Ursula' really been the victim. No, 'so are the rules, and that has to be tolerated'; that is what they all say in chorus. With those words any discussion, if there ever was one, generally ends.

> The German Constitution Article 1. 'The dignity of every human being is absolute. It is the duty of the state to protect and honour this dignity.'

In Germany this model of military induction was introduced during the rule of (the Victorian time) Emperor Wilhelm. Hitler happily carried on with the royal creation and today it is all business as usual - though, for the victims, worse than ever before. Of course, everything has a reason, and that goes for this area as well. Wilhelm and Adolf wanted obedient soldiers. Therefore independent people who might think for themselves were not welcome. For sure, they could still be used, but first they had to be changed to fit in: these civilians had to be properly trained, and I am not yet speaking about being trained in use of guns and grenades. No, before all that could even start they had to be shown that resistance is pointless, that there is no alternative to obeying orders and that they from now on are nothing but a bunch of nobodies.

So how do you achive all that in the quickest possible way? The answer was and is easy. The military medical induction, the musterung, is what is needed. Apart from the obvious purpose of declaring somebody reasonable fit for the service, this process is also good for something else: it is the first and very important step in turning a rebellious civilian into an obedient soldier. Yes, you won't need to beat anybody up to achive subservience: a military medical that is equal with forced nakedness will for sure do the trick.

Stripped in front of a draft commission and most anybody will learn to adapt; stripped by force in front of authoritarians and we will all feel worthless. If not before, when having to present one's genitals, pull one's foreskin back and spread one's buttocks for inspection, at least now the strongest of men will be small and weak - if not before, at least at this point the last resort of personal resistance will finally be gone. From now on the potential recruit will be well prepaired for the military training that is to come. Only in this way the very special military interest in testicles and foreskins can be understood.

In earlier times, in the 'Great' War's trenches, it might have been valuable for a soldier to have had such an induction to military life behind him. In the service of the Nazis probably the same. Having been dehumanised and removed of all dignity might have helped individual human beings in their transformation into a sick world of killing and maiming. That way one had left all civilisation and humanity back home. How else could you change peaceful citizens into soldiers fighting for Hitler and his cohorts?

However, times have changed. Modern European countries no longer aspire to expand their borders on behalf of their neighbours; our new leaders want to live in harmony with each other, and, for the first time ever, it seems like they are all taking these new vows of peace seriously. Allright, it might still be too early for all the armed forces to be abolished, but, at least, also they are now expected to adopt modern views on a broad scale. Not only are they expected not to encourage and teach rape and torture, they are also to live up to the principles of equality, humanity and respect for the individual within their own institutions. Correct, now also soldiers - on equal footing with other citizens - must be protected against violations of their basic human rights. Now also soldiers have a right to be treated with decency and respect.

All right, so what about the testicles, the foreskins and the backsides of the young men, conscripted or enlisted? Will these parts now be spared forced intrusion as well? No, unfortunately not. This area seems to be carefully exempted from protective reforms. The controls continue as usual, and for the victims it has changed for the worse not the better.

From being a perverted male-only ritual of 'initiation', the whole matter, the *musterung* (the military medical induction exam), in the name of so called 'equal rights' between the genders, has developed into nothing but a *state-approved* sexual humiliation process of young men. Today female medical inspectors, though themselves under no legal obligations neither to serve or to strip, have almost completely taken over the dominant roles in this age old humiliation process. Today these women have grabbed for themselves what could look like almost unlimited power over thousands of legally forced, naked young men.

As our ficticious Ursula felt, uncountable real life young men and big boys feel every day. A more perverted way of abusing the word 'equal rights' is difficult to imagine - and all this managed and regulated by a state in which obedience, nakedness, intimate examinations and submission in spite of all modern trends have never stopped mesmerizing those in power.

'Do I still have to go to musterung even if I volunteer to do civilian conscientious objector service? I am terrified about the musterung. I am only 16, but still, it is not that long before it will be my turn. Is it really true that they will put a finger up my bottom and that they will touch my penis?'

Rolf S.

Medical Rape

Giving Birth is a State Duty

In order to keep a people - a nation - alive men and women must work together. So, let us put all other 'minor' matters aside and have a look at the two great areas where the genders traditionally have had to do each their part in order for this to happen: men defend the home, if necessary with force; women carry and give birth to children. Without land and freedom men and women cannot live, and without children - who one day can take over - a nation obviously will die, will cease to exist.

To achieve the first objective men can, if necessary, be forced to take up arms. In many cases this is and must be acceptable. If the risk of being attacked is really there, a people must have a right to defend itself in order to survive. Even I, a life-long peace activist, can understand that and would volunteer to do my part. When it comes to the second thing, however, women are only *asked* and *encouraged* to do their duty. I can understand that as well. After all, one cannot legally force a woman to get pregnant. That would be an act not only totally in breach of international human rights but also in blatant contempt of what most people would regard as basic rights of dignity and privacy. At least that is how I look at such a prospect. But... could one really?

Some years ago I worked as a nurse in a hospice. In there at one point there was an old man who suffered from terminal cancer. He was an amiable, pleasant man, and, as soon as I had a spare moment, I was very happy to pop in and exchange some words with him. From this man I heard for the first time about a very special kind of forced medical exams. As a former senior civil servant in the entourage of the former Romanian dictator Ceausescu he knew, as I came to find out, quite a lot about this topic.

As most everywhere else, at least in the communist world, young men also in Romania, whether they wanted it or not, were called up for the armed forces. However, under the rule of Mr Ceausescu there was another kind of force as well. In his and his wife's maverick version of state communism also women were included in the common cause - to protect their country against the nasty capitalists. And, as mentioned above in the most fundamental example of job-sharing, they were to do it in their own way.

This is how it was thought to be: according to a 1966 Ceausescu plan, the Romanian population in the next thirty-four years should increase from twenty-three to thirty million citizens. And, in line with that pregnancy was made into just as big a patriotic duty for women as war service always had been for men. From now on contraceptives were forbidden, abortions outlawed and the production of children was made into a state priority. Of course, individual rights must give way to the rights of the state.... 'The foetus belongs to the society,' as Ceausescu expressed it himself. 'Every woman who avoids having children is a deserter.'

In order to make such a scheme work it indeed takes some innovative ideas. Just to encourage people to make more love will hardly do the trick. But, 'fortunately,' the people around the dictator knew what to do. One method was this one: with the help of regular compulsory gynaecological examinations the authorities would detect early pregnancies and this way at least prevent illegal abortions.

To be honest, I don't know how successful these examinations in reality were - at least not as long as we solely think in terms of increasing the number of pregnancies. About that the old man said nothing. Probably he didn't know himself - or maybe it wasn't even that important. In fact, another thing *was* achieved, and maybe *this* was what the whole thing really was about: the people as a whole was scared into submission. To remain childless was suspect and was seen as a deliberate unsocialist action - something every woman would try her best not to be accused of.

It is hard to believe but under Ceausescu (the communist darling of the western world) it was actually like that in Romania. I was shocked when I first time heard about it; it was an autumn day shortly before the death of this old man. Late that evening I sat there by his side, just as he once had sat by the side of the dictator. Now I heard repentance in his voice. 'No, one cannot do that. One cannot just order women to be gynaecologically examined just to make sure they fulfil their duties to the state to bear children. No, one cannot do that.' Together we thought it all through. Of course I agreed

Medical Rape

with him. Of course he was right in what he was saying. 'No, of course one cannot do that.'

About that conversation I have thought a lot ever since - about force in general and, more specifically, about people giving themselves forced access to other individuals' genitals. Of course, it is obvious to me: this must not happen. That is what one would call rape, isn't it? Yes, at least as long as we talk about Romania and this 'experiment' I am sure most people would quickly agree with me about that. But, so what about the forced examinations of genitals by the military in so many countries? That must go for the same, mustn't it? After all, conscripted and enlisted young people are human beings as well - at least as I see the world. Also these people must have a right to be protected against intrusions into their bodies. Just like the Romanian women should rightfully enjoy full rights to decide over their own bodies and private parts also here there must be limits for what state bodies can be allowed to do to people.

Indeed, there is a very good reason for being concerned about this matter. Why? Because not only a long dead dictator had his focus on other people's genitals, quite a few military bodies had and have as well: one of them, one in particular, is Germany's re-christened *Wehrmacht*, the *Bundeswehr* - the post-war German armed forces. In many ways these forces have distanced themselves from the past, but, when it comes to forcing themselves on to their enlisted and conscripted soldiers' genitals they haven't. In fact, sixty-five years after Hitler killed himself in the bunker they (i.e. their doctors) behave themselves in a more perverted way than ever before.

For me as a Swede and son of the European war generation it's all right that all able-bodied men in those days were 'requested' to help overcome the Nazis and their conscripted forces (those sacrificed on the altar of a criminal sake). But, to keep forcing young people to military (or civilian replacement) service sixty-five years later (when no enemy can be spotted no matter how hard one tries) that is to go too far. That goes for my native home land, where the conscription has only just been finally abolished, but it goes even so much more for the country that started both the world wars of the last century.

For them to continue on this path seems even more bizarre. After all, since the death of Hitler and since the end of the cold war there is no European country that needs to fear being attacked by any neighbouring state or by anybody else for that sake. To be honest who would for example try to conquer Germany? The Belgians? Or, maybe the Danes?

No it has all changed: the Romanians, as we have already seen, years ago stopped their forced pregnancy controls; the Russians suddenly lost their interest in converting us all into communists, and most west European states have dissolved their conscripted armed forces and made outdated ineffective mass armies into part of history. So it is that in most democratic countries nobody will be conscripted to march and nobody will against his will be 'asked' to present himself for a humiliating medical induction.

But, and there is a big but, there are some exemptions. For example: stubborn and intransigent power structures, especially in one central very powerful country, are still fighting for their places in the sun. Yes, precisely in the Federal State of Germany where once Hitler and his cohorts - helped and supported by loyal patriots - masterminded the biggest catastrophe the world has ever seen, precisely there obedient soldiers are still mass-produced for no other reason than for keeping officers and others in meaningless occupation. And, as nobody seems to have learned from the past, as usual the road to military obedience starts where it always used to start. For conscripts and enlisted men alike it all starts with checking so that the foreskin can be pulled back and forth without too much of an effort. No. nothing has changed when it comes to that part, at least not for the better.

Are military people really that concerned about young people's health as they obviously want us all to believe? Is that really what lies behind all this? No, of course not: it has nothing to do with health concerns; it is about power and obedience. Yes, more than anything else it is about making young people do what they are told. Being 'asked' to strip and spread one's buttocks can be a very effective start of a process in which a naturally rebellious youngster is changed into an non-questioning warrior.

Ceausescu's doctors checked Romania's vaginas to scare women away from birth control; Germany's doctors check foreskins in order to secure military obedience. As we soon will learn, in this modern example of continued oppression it seems like it is much more important that foreskins roll back and forth without problems than that coming soldiers have enough strength in arms and legs and that their lungs are sound enough for the hardship ahead.

'At several occasions I was examined stark naked by male and female doctors - without any screens but right there in front of young female assistants. Why such thorough checks have to be performed I have never understood, and nobody has ever explained it to me. At the time I felt deeply humiliated, and, thinking back, I still do. Today they - in order to hide the real reason for all this - explain it away as health service and medical screening. Seems odd, really. I don't think the French Napoleon-era soldiers, the first ones forced to strip, did that to allow the authorities to look for cancer.... No, there was another reason behind, and still there is.'

Julian H.

In the Shadow of the War

As I was still a small child back in my native Sweden my father told me stories from the war and, as something probably uncommon, also from his medical induction - that what the Germans call the '*musterung*'. He had stood there, as in those days was fully normal, stark naked in front of the induction officers and military doctors; completely unprotected he had 'discussed' his coming military service and his placements with these 'gentlemen'. This picture stayed with me during my whole childhood. It ruined my formative years. I was fully taken up by the anticipated humiliation, the one I knew was there to come. Yes, one day I would stand there myself. 'Take your head underneath your arm,' my father told me. This well-meant advice had saved himself, he claimed. By distancing himself from the body so to speak, he had helped himself to get through it all without too many scars on his soul. At least that was what he said. Father never had to fight in the war. There was a political reason for that which is too complicated to go into here and which also falls outside of the remit for this book. However, I can present you with a short version: Hitler chose to stop shortly before invading our country. Having had to fight or not, the war service stole years of my father's youth and when it came to certain things he knew what he was talking about.

'They will do with you what they want; it won't matter what you say. You will be their property. But, if you so to speak look at it all as a spectator from the outside, then you will have a good chance to survive unhurt.' That was what father told me, and that advice was to stay with me growing up: his words never lost their strangling grip on my early years.

Father had tried to protect me, but the knowledge of what was in store for me was in itself a catastrophe. The constant fear ruined my childhood.

Yes, it was clear to me: one day also I would have to become a soldier and the time there would start with standing naked in front of officers and doctors, all according to the principle that a boy as soon as he reaches adulthood has an innate duty to present himself as a piece of goods, a piece of state property.

Medical Rape

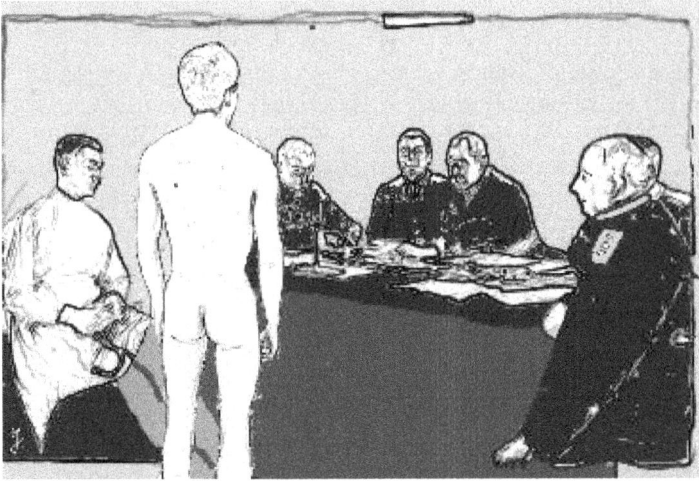

As said, already as a small child I knew what was in waiting, what one day also would happen to me. Apart from what father had told me there were other, though rare, indications regarding this very special initiation ceremony into male adulthood. At one time I also saw a film on television in which there was a *musterung* scene from around Edwardian time; the stage was Germany. There was a row of naked young men lined up in front of military doctors, all ready to be inspected in every detail - most likely with emphasis on their genitals - as preparation for their coming 'heroic' service in the 'Great' War's trenches.

WPflG § 15 Abs. 6 (The German Conscription Law) Male persons are from start of their 18th year of life subjects to this law.

What my father had told me and what the film had shown created the basis for what I would carry with me in the back of my head for the rest of my young years - this even if it, being a taboo, otherwise was never talked about. Precisely, this ritual of humiliation was never mentioned; it was a 'no go' area in everyday life - though it was for sure an 'all go' area for every young man in the country....

Musterung was the initiating process of growing into adulthood, but, though everything was known by everybody, it was still a subject carefully avoided. In public no man would ever admit he himself had had to stand there as God, or whoever he believed in, had created him. Those who already *had* served king and country, they talked about cruel officers, they talked about the stupidity of blind obedience, but, funny enough, they hardly ever talked about the day it all began. If anybody ever did, it was all made completely harmless. 'Oh, that? That's just a ritual, something natural; it's part of it,' and 'it just took a minute'.

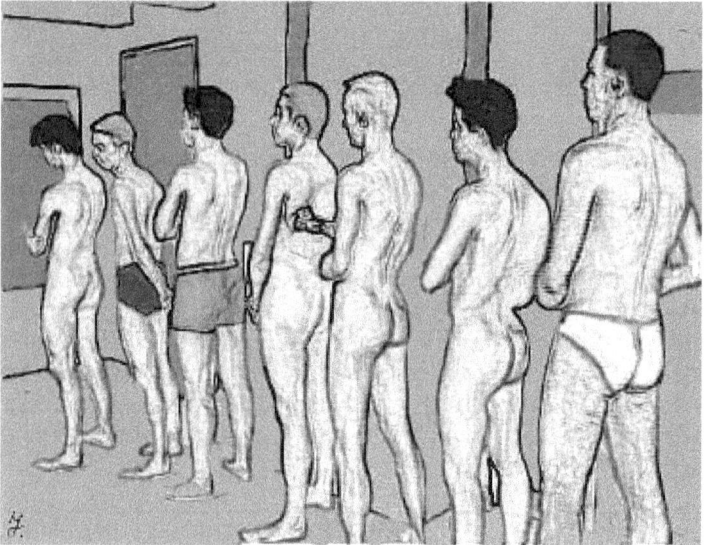

When the day finally came, I happened to be lucky. Time had changed, and it was no longer as in my father's days. The year was 1969; we were at the height of the cold war, and the Soviet Union was just across the Baltic. But, it was no longer as I had expected it to be. Two days the procedure was to take, and it was all very modern, actually like a high-tech gym. A number of psychological and physical tests were to be performed, and people were friendly and professional. Apart from the underlying obligatory nature of the whole procedure it wasn't actually too bad.

Medical Rape

At one point I also had to attend a medical examination. Also this man was friendly, and it was all very quick - probably a matter of three or four minutes. At the end he had asked me, positioned on a couch, to pull down the pants. A quick examination of the groin followed, and thereafter it was all over. I found nothing embarrassing with that; there was nothing humiliating about it. Only the fact I wasn't there as a volunteer was for me a problem - as it would be for any person who values his freedom.

It is now forty years since my *musterung.* As it wasn't that bad, why do I then still remember this event so clearly? At the same time I have no recollection whatsoever of the dental appointment I must have had the same year? Most likely, that must have been physically more painful. However, it had had nothing to do with removal of my freedom, with stripping. I had gone there myself; it had all been my own decision. The state hadn't asked for a check up of my teeth: I had. By the *musterung* it was different. I had never asked anybody to check my private parts - no matter if friendly or not. Ultimately, that is what it is all about; it is about honour and respect for the personal boundaries of (what you at least would like to call) free human beings. It is about being allowed to make one's own decisions about one's own body.

However, by the military there is no space for such extra-ordinary luxury. All right, I might have had some initial luck, but soon the real nature of the whole institution would re-affirm itself: from the day I finally was called up for service my body no longer belonged to me but to the state, and the result of that would soon be obvious. Just as father once had said, now they could do with me what they wanted, and this they did. Yes, by the *musterung* I had been lucky (and if that had not been the case I would never have had the courage to write this story), but a legal right to be treated with respect for my own person, that I did no longer have. That respect, which most people in democratic countries would take for granted, disappeared in the same moment I entered through the gate. In the boot camp I would be humiliated and have my human dignity ruined in the same way as has happened to so many millions of other young men both before and after. While teaching me how to help defend my own people's freedom

19

and dignity, they, the same people, assisted by their stripes and chevrons-decorated helpers, robbed me of my own.

Especially *forced* military training must be mentally damaging for the individual. I was quickly convinced about that. All right, I followed my father's advice; I tried to 'put my head under the arm', and by doing so at least I thought I would save myself.

But no, to be honest, that method doesn't work. Nobody returns undamaged from such a place. I felt it with myself already at the time, and how right I was in general terms I came to realise years later as I worked in a psychiatric unit under the Danish Ministry of Defence. Yes, in fact, such a unit existed, a place for (mainly) conscripts who had broken down mentally while serving in the armed forces. They were 'sent in to the lunatics' as it was said - a term that was generally used within the forces in order to scare young people away from seeking this 'easy' way out.

During my work at this place I came across quite a few astonishing stories, but more than anything else I was struck by an individual case which made me realise what a madhouse this really was - not because of the admitted young victims themselves but because of the simple fact that the (now post cold war) modern society could allow this place its very existence: what an insane idea.

Yes, I was rather shocked, as I realised what was being done to eighteen-year-old Jens. Believe it or not, he had been sentenced to prison for having asked a friend to break his leg (Jens's own). By having that done, he thought he could avoid a part of the service he feared. But there was something Jens had not calculated with: by doing so he actually harmed state property (i.e. his own leg), and for this the young man was sent down by the court....

All this is now long ago, but still, it has never gone away. Even today I am unable to free myself from the strangle grip of the military. I cannot run away from it. It is always there with me. I might be a lucky man after all: I never ended under a white cross; I wasn't humiliated by the *musterung*, and my daily life isn't really completely ruined either. No, there are good things in my life as well.

For millions of other young people both before and after me it was and is different: they had and have to suffer the

Medical Rape

insufferable; they had and have to endure the unendurable. So it was, and, obviously, so it stays. There seems to be no end to this military madness of mental destruction. And, as we have understood of all this, you actually don't have to fight wars to feel the brunt of this system that itself, so to speak, was built up with only one purpose - to destroy what others had built up, both in life and property. No, also those who never had to fight, those who never had to risk their lives on the battlefield, those who never had to see destruction and massacres, they can still belong to the millions of people whose lives are ruined for ever after.

'What is absolutely unbelievable is that these examinations are also performed during and at the end of the service. Great isn't it? What business can it be for the army the whole time to check foreskins and backsides of people? A normal person is not exposed to that at his work place. I think this is a downright disgrace. I don't want my friend to be examined in such a way. That it shouldn't be enjoyable for the secretaries to watch, don't try and tell me that, please.

'Last year my friend (who is an enlisted soldier) was examined by an army doctor as he had a bad cold. The doctor gave him some medication, and, at the end of the consultation, he was asked to pull down his trousers so that it could be made certain everything was 'as it should'. Thereafter the doctor touched his genitals. What business of his was that? After all, he consulted for a cold....'

Angela S.

Lars G Petersson

My Neighbour's Son

Some years ago a female acquaintance of mine - sexologist and psychiatrist with expertise in treatment of victims of torture - in the course of a discussion suddenly asked the question: 'how can it be that soldiers when ordered to rape actually get an erection? One must feel lust for that, or?' Yes, that was a good question, asked by somebody who in fact should have been the expert on the subject but still wasn't. In fact, how could she be? After all, nobody with first-hand knowledge would ever truthfully answer that question, leaving her, excluded by nature from having her own experiences, with an unanswered enigma. Today I think I know the answer. Sexual arousal is not entirely limited to a loving sexual relationship if anyone has ever thought it was. There is a darker side to that part of life as well - even if it for most people would constitute a taboo, an absolute no-go-area, even just to talk about it.

Suffered humiliation and subservience can not only cause shame and suffering but can also evoke sexual lust. The consequence can be an erection. If not wanted, this can be a very shameful situation for a man to find himself in - a situation better quickly forgotten, better never talked about and, for sure, better prevented from ever happening again. However, the day when a humiliated person, who got aroused by the event, could change from being the victim into taking on the part of the perpetrator must not necessary be that far away. The change can come faster than we would ever wish to think.

Fortunately, under normal circumstance it might never go that far. But, that is nothing self evident. Subservience, sexual humiliation and powerlessness, or the opposite of that, no matter what role the individual plays, victim or perpetrator, it can all provoke sexual feelings of lust. And, horrible truth, nothing is permanent.... Today a person might be the victim, tomorrow he/she might feel pleasure in dominating and humiliating others. When somebody in such a way gets aroused when humiliating others, then the target (some would say) has been reached. Of course, such a person is not desired in a peaceful society: for aggressive warmongering forces, however, it is something else. For them this state of the mind can indeed be helpful.

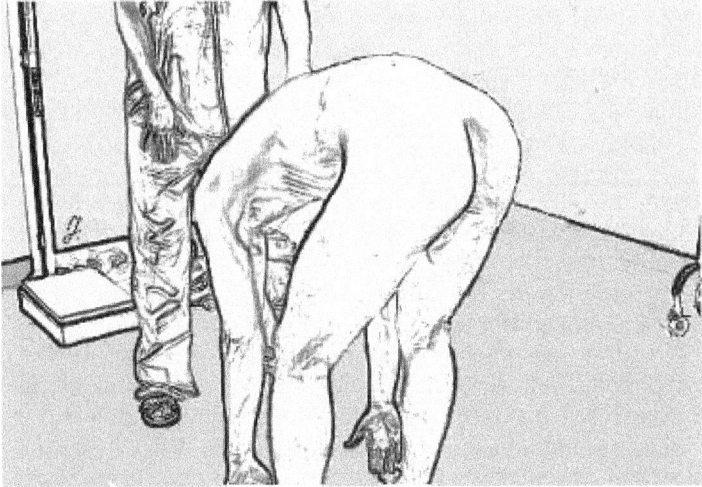

In the same way as the child that has been exposed to incest can evolve into a perpetrator himself, so can the victim of humiliation and abuse turn into a war criminal - a torturer. The humiliating *musterung,* with its built in sexual harassment, can very well be the first step in this direction - all in line with the principle: 'when my own dignity is gone, the road can open up to do to others what once was done to me.' In many armed forces so it was and so it still is.

'As I started to recall all the details, it was clear that it was the examination of my private parts which had left permanent scars in my soul. I am now constantly angry, but I am unable to talk about it. I am simply too ashamed, though I have done nothing wrong. The whole matter has in a way started to devour me from within. It is there in my head all the time.'

Burkhard M.

Today it is well known that if the right methods are used almost every human being can be changed into a torturer. There are numerous examples telling this story. The most famous is likely to be what happened during the nineteen sixties dictatorship in Greece. Specific circumstances led to that fame: during the reign of the Papadopoulos Junta effective methods in this field were not just used, as they were so many other places and still are, they were studied and observed by outsiders. Later even a book and a film were made. *'My Neighbour's Son'* they were both called, and it was all about how individuals can be turned into torturers.

Spring 2010. According to the military authorities themselves three recruits with the 'General Field Marshall Rommel's armoured brigade' have been harassed, beaten up and probably mistreated sexually by some of the other conscripted soldiers.

Oh, that was interesting... and shocking. How could that happen? And, why does such abuse often happen in military but almost never in civilian settings? Could it be because of the vicious circle we just talked about? Could it be that the victims-turned-perpetrators theory here again has shown its true, ugly face? I think it is very likely so.

Apart from the horrible attacks on these young men isn't it also remarkable that a Hitler-era field marshal like Mr Rommel still, sixty-five years after the disastrous war of aggression, is honoured with having a military institution named after him... In fact it is. But, that's another story.

The shocking realisation: almost every human being can be changed into one.... What is needed is dependence, humiliation, punishment, insecurity, subordination and maybe some other ingredients from the same shelf. After somebody has been humiliated and beaten long enough you show him how he can swap roles. The victim turns into a perpetrator; the torturer is ready for action. What before was impermissible and perverted now feels 'normal'; the abused has turned into the abuser; the one being used has become the user.

There is no natural law saying that built up hate necessarily must be channelled back on to the people who once were the oppressors. Hate can be projected on to others as well, and it might be 'easier', 'safer' and more common to do so. After all, 'someone' just has to pay. If it cannot be the harasser him/herself, so what about somebody who belongs to the same

Medical Rape

sort of group - the same race, nationality or gender? Or maybe somebody with the same or similar political views? Or, why not just anybody?

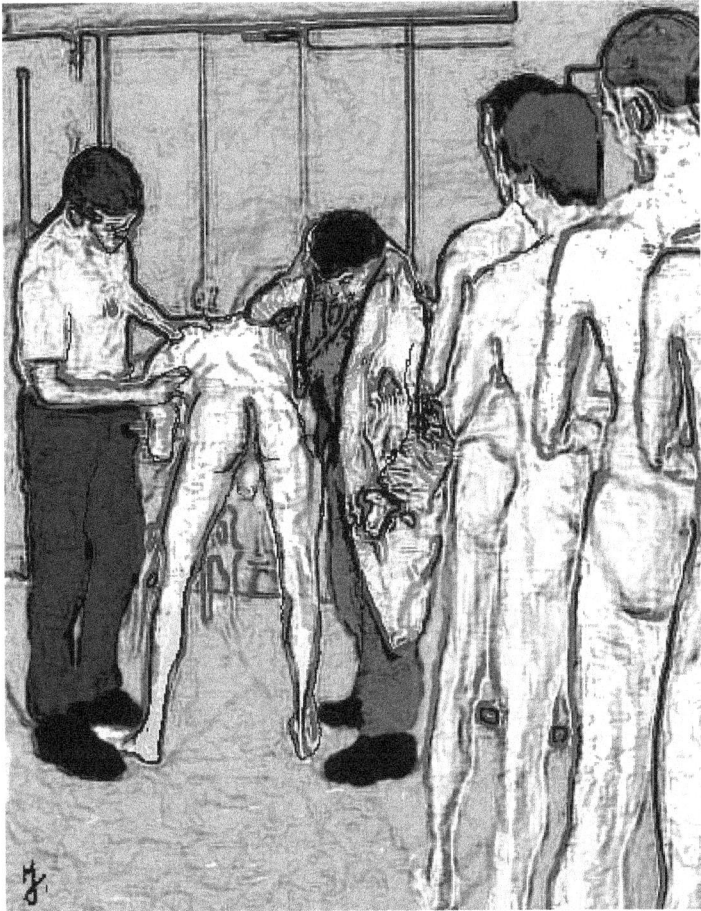

Now the change in personality has happened; according to this recipe it could very well be your own son, or maybe your daughter, who has changed into an abuser or, forbid it, a torturer. Yes, it could in fact be anyone of us: it could be you or I; it could be uncle John or aunt Phyllis. Nobody could be sure they would be exempted. They might say so themselves, but first being in the situation will actually tell.

Examples of this are plentiful. To make it short: the hate against the guilty can spread to others. This way racism and xenophobia can develop, as can hate against the opposite gender. The hate spreads to all those who fit into the picture. In this way a torturer comes into being. Now he will do what he before would have found impossible. He will do what he is told, and, what is even worse, he might even feel pleasure in doing it. Having once been humiliated, he now feels pleasure when doing the same to others. And, remember, 'he' might very well be a 'she'. There is no gender monopoly on cruelty.

The first time I realised this about the human nature I was horrified. In fact, I still am. More so while it sometimes seems like nothing can be done about it. The Greek dictatorship was short-lived; it is now part of history, but the methods which were used by these people they live on and they thrive. They thrive in dictatorial and warmongering states, but they are, in moderate versions, also to be found most everywhere else, also in Europe. Odd really, as the mentally ruined person, the brain washed machine, is no longer requested in this post Hitler continent. Be it so or not, someone must have forgotten to cancel the delivery the day the product wasn't needed any-more....

When it comes to the German military medicals we have a sad example of how something instead of being radically changed with modern times has not just stayed on as it was but in fact got worse.

This is the sad background for the fact that young men from age seventeen and upwards, ever since the late sixties, in special conscription centres, by the armed forces and by the civilian authorities responsible for replacement work for conscientious objectors have been paraded naked in front of female medical inspectors and their likewise female as-sistants. Yes, that's the reason for why they have been para-ded in front of those who are not themselves - due to being females - subjects to the conscription law. They have been paraded as cattle on a market place, and all that has been part of an extreme way of interpreting the concept 'equal rights between the genders at work'.

Medical Rape

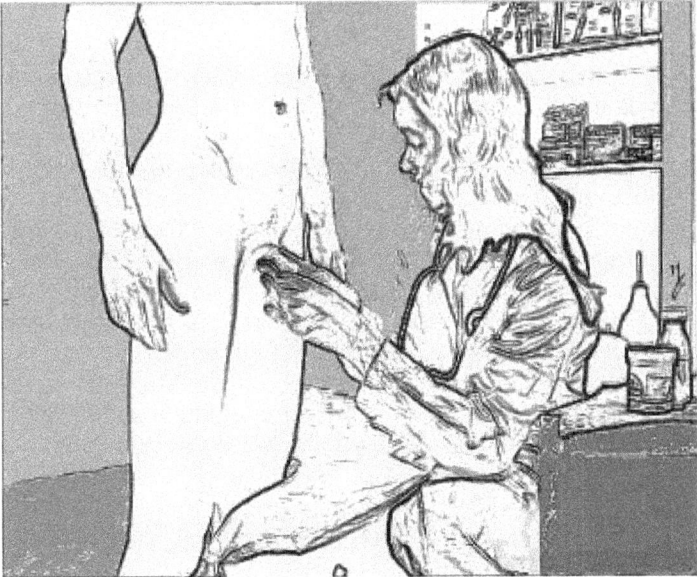

'This is a situation that I would declare as the first step in an extreme process of humiliation. This is what I would state is a practice which can lead to very serious consequences, and, forgive me for saying so, this I would say is a degrading treatment of other human beings that unwillingly will lead my thoughts back to times and places which none of us today wants to be associated with....

I'm Anxious

Also I was once a small anxious child. Today there are numerous others. They all wait for the day of the great strip, for the
day when their state will inspect them and assess their 'ability'. Then, after it is all over, they will continue to think about it
till the end of their life.

It is not long ago since I read following on a German internet
site: 'I am seventeen. On Wednesday I have to go to *musterung,* and I don't know what to do. I have heard so much
about having to pull down the trousers and expose myself.
Can that anyhow be avoided? I am not happy to say so, but I
have a very small penis (3-4cm), and it would be extremely
embarrassing for me to show myself to others like that. What
can I do.' Tim.

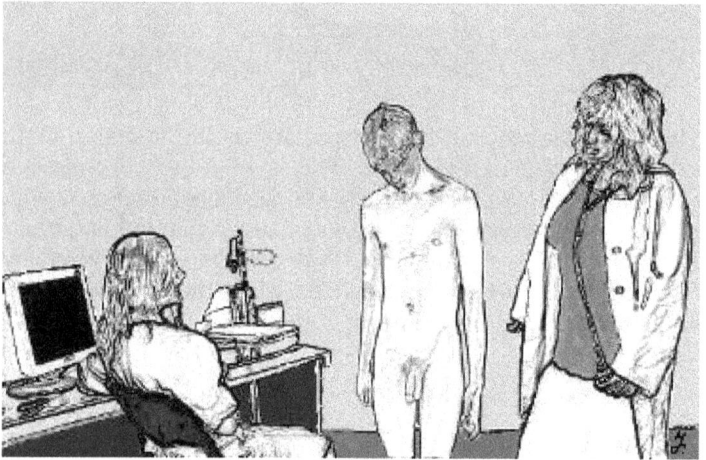

That was an anonymous cry for help on the internet. To me it
sounded like a cry in the dark night. Many must have 'heard'
Tim's virtual cry of distress, still nobody could have known
from where it came. And, even if we had known, what could
we have done to help this distressed young man? What could
we have told him? To be honest, not much. Maybe only
something like this: 'Tim, you are now seventeen; soon you
will turn eighteen. From now on your body belongs to the
state and its representatives, and - just as when you have

bought something yourself - now they want to check out their property. Fair, isn't it? They want to see if it all works.'

Yes, it's correct, even if Tim - according to international law - is still a child and, in line with German legislation, this far has not been given a right to vote, he is already subject to the so called *Wehrüberwachung* (law governing male German citizens' duty to serve their country) with strictly limited rights of freedom for the individual person.

In a 'democratic' way grown up people have decided it all for him. Smart isn't it? In order for Tim to protect the freedom of his country they have prescribed to remove his own... and he himself was never asked. In fact a strange thing really - and completely contradictory.

From now on Tim has to learn blind obedience, and, as first lesson in that process, he must pull down his pants and show his penis, testicles and anus. That is the first step in teaching him to become a soldier. In fact it's a matter of getting used to it, isn't it? And, be sure of that, as soon as it has been done for the first time the sense of having a private sphere to defend and protect at least should be partly gone, making it all so much more easy. A few more times and there is no privacy left - play can start. Yes, this is of course all so because of a very special reason: thereafter it will be so much more easy to teach him what it's really all about - shooting, marching, killing and, if necessary, sacrificing his life for the state.

After all, this process is nothing new. In fact, for years that's the way things have been. 'No Tim, you are not the only one who has had to walk this path. You are just one in a long, long row. At the *musterung* you are not allowed to hide yourself; you have to present yourself. Nakedness is here the method, and, to be honest, it cannot be that bad, can it? After all, contrary to your fears, the size of the penis will not be measured. You can rest assured about that. It might be that they will smile at it, but more it won't be. Tim you must have understanding for that. To be honest, even if you haven't, it doesn't really matter; you still have to accept what is to be done to you. That they have written very clearly in the law book, and not least in all their rules and regulations.'

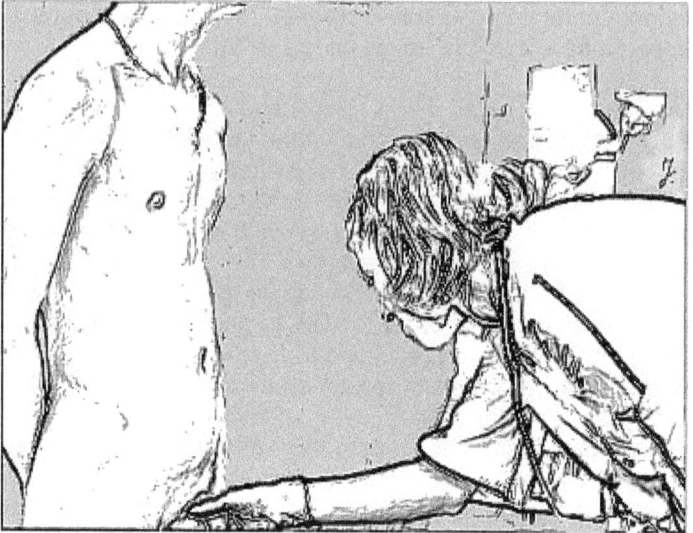

To be honest, also I ask myself why the penis can be of such an interest for the *Bundeswehr*, the German armed forces. Not the size of it but especially the function of the foreskin. Funny actually, or is it really? I have asked all responsible authorities in the country; I have asked all members of the Parliament (yes all of them, both before and after the election); I have asked the so called *Wehrbeauftragten,* a kind of parliamentary ombudsman for all soldiers; and, not least, I have asked most of the medical boards in the country (all those at state level as well as the federal umbrella organisation). All these and of course also the ministers and ministries of health and defence, have heard my questions. They have all been asked for their opinion.

However, nobody, absolute nobody, can, will or is able to give me a proper answer. They all remain silent or hide behind jargon or gobbledegook. In fact, it seems like they haven't got a clue what else to do. Of course, they all know they are wrong, but they also know they are not allowed to say so. The easy way out: pass the buck, put the head into the sand, and hope it will all go away.

Why blame them for trying this? After all, it has always worked before. Nobody would ever speak out - not those in political power, and, to be honest, definitely not the general public.

Medical Rape

Though all men in the German speaking world would know what this is all about, though they might be raging in private, few of them would do anything seriously about it. It will normally end there; the personal shame is too big for anything beyond writing a few anonymous e-mails. Yes, it ends with a tight fist in the pocket (happy as they are that they now at least can keep their own trousers on). The soup box seems to be no alternative.

For those deeply responsible for these acts of state legitimated sexual abuse this speechlessness on behalf of the general public is indeed fortunate. Only due to this national state of silence these members of the medical profession and their willing helpers - all those performing these institutionalised acts of mental rape - have for so long been left completely in peace with whatever they have been up to.

For many years they shared this luck with misbehaving perverts within the Catholic Church. Those clerics where also for a very long time protected both by their victims' silence and the general aversion to touch the issue even with the longest of barge-poles. No, just as little as anybody volunteered to address *that* issue before the gate finally burst open, every effort has been made to stay out of *this* discussion.

Franz Josef Jung was at the time of research for this book German minister of defence. Today his successor's name is Karl-Theodor Freiherr zu Guttenberg. Both were once, like all others, *mustered* stark naked. Both had their genitals thoroughly inspected and controlled. For me there is no doubt that the young Franz Josef and the young Karl-Theodor were embarrassed and enraged about being treated like that - though it probably was still among males only. Dr. Jung and Dr. zu Guttenberg, however, have both lost the courage to speak out now when they have their chance and would be heard.

> 'I stood there naked in front of people who were totally indifferent to the fact that I was deeply hurt. And, what was even worse: it was all state-approved and legalised. I was not ill, and it was not about health screening. No, it was an ability test for war duty.'
>
> Marius D.

Dieter Speaks Out

'When you are eighteen you think about freedom and inde-
pendence. Especially at this point to be forced by women to
strip and have the foreskin inspected and controlled, pulled
back and forth, that I found extremely humiliating,' Dieter, a
friend of mine, suddenly said, just like that, out in the blue.
Before that day he had never talked to anybody about this
subject, about what they did to him back then, he continued to
tell me, and I am sure he was right about that. Between us at
least it had never been a topic.

It was all quite odd really. It was as if Dieter all of a sudden
just had woken up. At the same time it appeared to me as if
he wasn't fully aware of the fact that he now had broken the
ice and spoken out loud what had obviously been on his mind
years on end. Yes, it might not have been intentional, but still,
now it had happened: he had allowed me to enter his secret
world of intense suffering.

From now on there was no return, and Dieter had more to
tell. 'Of course, when you are examined this way you just
want to sink through the floor. One is very little in there. I
wouldn't allow just anybody to touch my private parts, but in
there they just take it for granted; they don't ask for your
permission. To have to turn around and bend forward almost
felt like a relief, as I at that moment at least were free of eye
contact.

'On top of that she wanted to know, while she had a look at
my penis, if I had any problems with peeing (of course not)
and if the foreskin could be pulled back all the way (of
course it can). Obviously she didn't trust my answer but tested it herself anyway.

'After she had thoroughly inspected this part for a while, I
was asked to turn and bend forward while she pulled apart
my buttocks. At that moment I thought, now it comes, the
finger, but nothing happened. She must have looked for a
few seconds; after that I was allowed to pull back on my
underpants and follow her to the desk. There the secretary
waited - with a smirk on her face.'

Thomas H.

Medical Rape

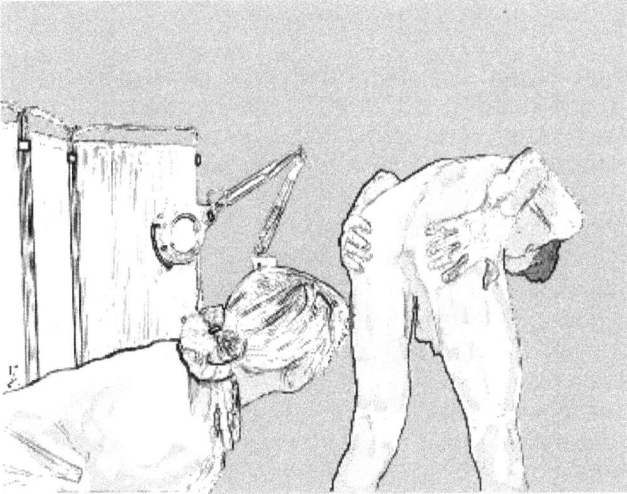

Today Dieter thinks that the medical induction, the *musterung*, is only the first (but immensely important) step in the process of forcing young people into submission - to break their resistance. I can only agree. Also others must ask themselves the question: can this really be part of modern Germany, or shouldn't it rather be banned to the history books? As Emperor Wilhelm and later Adolf Hitler were still around it was for sure all about terror and show of power. The strip examinations were important parts of the process of converting civilians into obedient soldiers. Thereafter, however, our understanding of the role of armed forces in modern society all over Europe has changed. Not least human rights and human dignity have been allowed to be (at least) considered. So it has been also in post-war, post-Nazi Germany.

> 'As the doctor starts to examine the private parts she will request the foreskin to be pulled back. Most of the youngsters will now be fairly stressed, as all eyes focus on their willies. But, if someone at this point hesitate to long or start to shake, he can rest assured the doc will do it herself. And, if that happens, it will go right back....'
>
> Secretary Melanie U.

Lars G Petersson

Forgetful Regulators and Bureaucrats

German authorities just love their rules and regulations. Therefore it is indeed odd that they, when it comes to this case,
do not even seem to follow their own ones. Can it really be
true that they exactly here have forgotten most everything
they have written themselves?

In the conscription law, paragraph 17, it is clearly said that
the medical examination exclusively shall be about the
individual young person's strict ability to train as a soldier - to
learn how to defend the country, nothing but that. There is no
word there about cancer prevention or problems with foreskins, nothing of the sort. No, the law says that all males from
age seventeen are to be examined in order to establish
whether their standard of health makes them *able or disable
to serve in the country's armed forces*. It continues to establish that these young people are obliged to make themselves
available for such examinations, and it stresses that *'such
examinations which according to medical science are
considered necessary for making such a decision are to be
performed'*.

There it is: according to the conscription law itself the medical examination is exclusively about deciding whether or not a
person *is able for armed service*, nothing but that. It has, or
shouldn't have, anything to do with anything else. It has absolutely nothing to do with preventive medicine or health
screenings.

On top of this, as basis for the medical selecting process of
future soldier, conscripts and enlisted staff, the Ministry of
Defence has created a list of requirements, the so called *'Tä-
tigkeitskatalog'*. The twenty specific requirements which are
listed here are seen as the minimum standards for somebody
who should be seen able to fulfil basic military training as a
soldier by the German *Bundeswehr.* Interesting but not surprising: nowhere in this list there is any talk whatsoever about
examinations of genitals or peoples backsides - not a word
about that. After all, why should there be?

Medical Rape

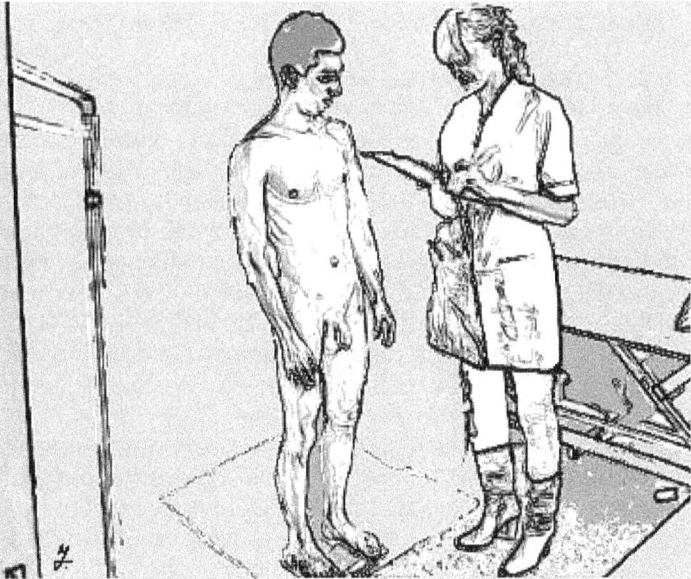

There are good reasons to reflect over this whole matter. In fact, what *is* it really about? Would we for example talk about female candidates - all of them of course volunteers - then there would be no such examinations to consider or discuss. Confused? No need to be. Let's have a close look into the rule book.

The armed forces also have other instructions which should be followed by their doctors, and reading them leads us on to something rather extraordinary. These instructions, the so called *ZDv,* the 'central service instructions', clarify in every detail how to examine *male* genitals. However, when it comes to the *female* counterparts just as clear orders are given that 'an examination of genitals shall not be included', but,' instead of that, a (gynaecological) history shall be taken following a prepared form'. Only in case of special medical concerns a gynaecological examination, according to this text, is to be performed. And, if so, the person will be referred to a consultant in gynaecology (by the her own choice).

In fact, this seems to be a very good and reasonable practice. But, if so, why are men not treated in the same sensible and professional way? The answer is simple: if this was exclusively about medicine, then that's the way it would have been. But, it isn't. There are other factors involved here as well and that's what makes the difference.

The forced intimate examination of (male) soldiers (both conscripts and enlisted) is a traditional part of military medicine, or, as we have seen, a part of the 'training'. However, with the introduction of female warriors there was no chance one could continue as usual. Some adjustments had to be made. Otherwise two obvious things would immediately have happened: a major sex scandal would have hit the headlines (WOMEN SEXUALLY ABUSED BY MILITARY PERVERTS) in bigger writing than the announcement of a third world war, and there would have been no woman candidates left to harm: they would all have been gone.

Therefore the continued abuse of men is allowed to keep up the traditions (as few people would be bothered about that) while women are protected against the same by modern laws and ideas of human dignity (this way keeping the perverts away from the headlines). What a splendid idea!

'Let me be frank: it felt like an outright assault - it was like someone breaking into my soul, into the innermost of my identity. In this country there must be so many wounded souls walking around. They must be many more than we are able to imagine. In any case, I am one of them. All right, my *musterung* was years ago, but I will probably never be able to leave the humiliating experience behind me.'

Werner G.

Medical Rape

Unexpected Help

As the German Ministry of Defence goes to great length to defend their very special medical checks and to declare them as nothing but just a commendable contribution to the general public-health service they are not completely alone. In fact, they get welcome help in that mission by nobody less than a well known professor of andrology. For a reason difficult to comprehend, this man, Eberhard Nieschlag, has established himself as a stern advocate for status quo - because, as he puts it, 'there is no equivalent health offer for men as the one there is for women'. And, he doesn't stop with that: to the delight of the establishment he goes on to declare that 'the ministry of defence therefor plays an important role in detecting cancer by young men'.

That was indeed unexpected help from the civilan sector of the public health service. The minister of defence must be very pleased. But, why has this man established himself as a military lobbyist? What could be his real motive? Could it be that another interest than pure concern for the patients is playing a leading role in all this? In fact, it's not the first time a civilian expert has been used to boost military establishments' credibility when their own arguments and qualifications have fallen short of doing the job.

No matter what, if somebody wants to be seen as an expert he/she needs to have not only the necessary theoretical qualification but also a relevant background in the specific subject that is being addressed. As a professor of andrology Dr Nieschlag has that, hasn't he? To be honest, I am not quite convinced, though I might be proved wrong. In fact, my research into Dr Nieschlag's background has told me that he is an internationally renowned expert in *reproductive* medicine. He is working (unfortunately still unsuccessfully) on the invention of a pill for the man.

However, with urological screening he has for me no known background. So, on what research is this professor relying when he speaks out in favour of the controversial *musterung* examinations of young people's private parts? Could it be a study published in two parts by Römer et al.? The first, *'Früherkennung von Hodentumoren - Musterung als Prävention'* (Screening for Testicular Tumours - *Musterung* as Prevention), appeared in the October 2001 edition of the German journal for military medicin *'Wehrmedizin und Wehrpharmazie'* (Military Medicin and Pharmaceutics**),** and the second, *'Akzeptanz und Ergebnisse der Hodentastuntersuchung anlässlich der Musterung'* (Acceptance and Conclusions from Examinations of the Testicles at the *Musterung*), followed in the August/September 2003 edition of the same journal.

If so, then I have some serious concerns. Uncritically to accept information from this specific study, which, for whatever reason, tried to establish the *musterung* examinations as an excellent way to detect cancer (disregarding all the extremely serious short and long term implications of the whole procedure) would indeed be alarming. It would be so not least because of the nature of the articles themselves but also because of the background of the authors. None of them are experts in what they are here talking about. When knowing how much this study has been relied on by those fervently protecting the examinations, this is indeed remarkable - and shocking.

No doubt, after learning all that, there are quite a few questions which need to be asked. For example: why did a famous professor allow himself to rely on such questionable research? And, why did he lend his name to that sort of lobbying? I am sure that Dr Nieschlag, a medical person trained 'never to use the medical art contrary to the basic commandments of humanity' and 'to practise the profession with consciousness and dignity', did not intentionally defend the forced humiliating examinations of naked youngsters as such, but, if not, why did he not give the consequences of his support a second thought? After all, why did he not know what it's all about? And, finally, if this man really wanted to lobby for male health screening, why didn't he instead start a campaign in favour of one based on regularity and free choice, precisely in line with what is being offered women?

Yes, why did he not start to speak out for regular checks, either by self examination or by a doctor of one's own choice, or both? After all, as an andrologist he should know that this disease very well can strike long after the armed forces has loosen its grip on the young individual. The danger is not limited to a year or two around the time a person might serve in the forces or as a conscientious objector. There is no need

to be a professor of andrology to know that. And, there is no
need to be a psychologist to realise that a person suffering
from the mental scars of humiliating medical 'examinations'
only very reluctantly ever will go back for more of the same.
No, that person won't give 'them' another chance.

The result can be an early death. That is why it is so important that young people are treated with respect and dignity
and not scared away from health care for life.

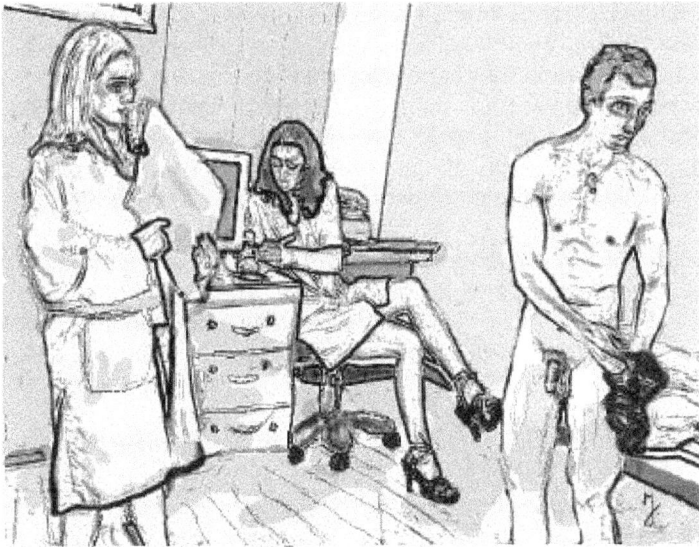

'That's absurd! Preposterous!' Dieter, my old friend from before, said as I told him about the professor's idea. 'What they do
there has nothing to do with health care. That's just a cover.
It's a sex game for perverts.'

That female assistants had been present, Dieter found extremely difficult. 'I was so embarrassed as I stood there in front
of them. And worst of it all, the whole situation, the complete
exposure, aroused me sexually - after all, I was hardly more
than a boy.' It might be a complete, total, massive taboo, but
this is human reality: before this day Dieter had never been in
a sexual relationship; to be naked in the presence of women,
no matter the circumstances, was altogether new to him. He
had no chance to 'decide the outcome', and therefore, left

with no (garment) protection, the road to the ultimate male humiliation and embarrassment had been left for him wide open.

'This was no surprise for me. Long time before I had to go there, I started to fear getting an erection. And, as it turned out, it did happen. I tell you, it was extremely embarrassing to stand like that in front of these women. Today I am very angry about it. And, it torments me to think that they, the doctor and her assistant, actually enjoyed seeing me like that, stripped and totally left to their mercy.'

Indeed, strange human nature: enjoyment for one part and hell for the other. As Dieter now says to me: 'it feels like I have been raped. I cannot stop thinking about it. Sometimes, when it's really bad, then I think about committing suicide, about making an end to it all. To call that kind of medical abuse "a serious health care offer on level with what is offered to women", as that professor did, is nothing but a mockery.'

'It is indeed amazing to observe the eagerness they show when checking penises in the army. They do it when you come and go, and they do it in between. How can it be that precisely these people, those working for an institution built up to kill, are so interested in precisely this organ - the one not made to terminate but in fact to start life?'

Michael K.

Dieter was the person who first introduced me to this strange German world of state sanctioned perversion. He volunteered without being asked. After that I started to look for other victims, and there was no problem finding them. I discovered a world of shame, escape from the past and, not least, a world of anger and resentment. It has indeed shocked me that so many men suffer a whole long life due to perverted medicine. However, I am not surprised.

Medical Rape

A Rendezvous in Cafe Adler

'Back then I repeatedly had to go through all that nonsense,' Sebastian K. told me as we, in the course of my research for this book, met in Cafe Adler, the famous cold war meeting point close to the now disappeared Checkpoint Charlie in Berlin. 'For me it was the most embarrassing and humiliating experience I have ever in my life had to endure. I felt deeply hurt in my human dignity and had no idea how to help myself while it took place. At that time, only aged seventeen, I did not have the necessary courage to open my mouth and just say NO.'

In the time directly after meeting the people from the military 'health service', Sebastian had huge problems with his self esteem. He turned to self harm, started to cut himself - all of that, as he sees it now, a desperate attempt to 'have something that just belonged to him'. After all, they had taken everything else away from him. 'There is a scar on my private parts which I will never show to anybody. It's mine only.'

Then years passed by and by chance, four years ago, Sebastian, while surfing the internet, discovered stories told by other men which showed close resemblance to his own experiences. At this point it was clear to Sebastian that he wasn't alone in his suffering. There were many others out there who felt the same. What he this far desperately had tried to forget could no longer be hidden away.

'Within myself a feeling of deep humiliation became paramount. After all these years it all became clear to me what had constantly been haunting my soul, had I been aware of it or not. From now on it was all out there in the open, and it would never again let go. Today only sport activities (for short periods of time) can divert my thoughts and subdue the aggressive feelings which now have completely absorbed my mind. When I have worked out very hard I feel a bit better, but the effect won't last; very soon it's all back with me. It's all a constant fight against an overwhelming enemy.

'I have tried most anything to come to terms with this demon. On and off I also let my anger out against fictive computer enemies in so called *'ego-shooter'* games. But nothing of it is to much avail. It' all there with me from early morning till late night. And, it won't even stop there: in the last couple of years

I have been suffering from horrible dreams. In the dreams I am surrounded by people dressed in white - and I am naked; I am unable to protect myself. Most every morning I then wake up early, long before day starts, soaked in sweat and with only one word in my head: *musterung*. I am completely unable to let it go. It keeps feeling like if I am back in the situation. I keep thinking about the young women who were present as it happened.

'Growing older I have come to realise that my whole sexuality must have been influenced by what happened. I cannot find sexual satisfaction with a woman, but only by helping myself. I don't exaggerate when I say I suffer. Every day I suffer, and there seems to be no end to it.'

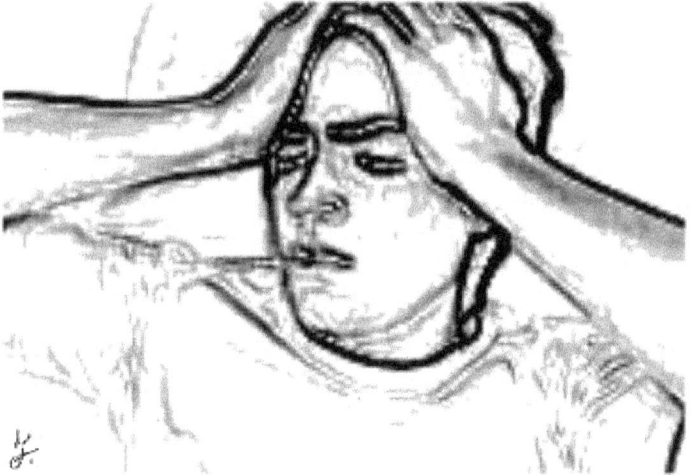

Thereafter Sebastian repeatedly has informed the authorities about his private and intimate problems. He has told them in detail what happened and what consequences it has had for him. But, of course, all to no avail - not even a worthless reply he has received as response to his very private letters, not one single one, absolutely nothing.

'And, who can allow himself to say I am a coward? If so, he should see what I have done to myself. He should see the scars on my very private parts, those I have inflicted on myself.'

Medical Rape

Sebastian suffers, and I ask myself why his county has done all that to him. Why on earth was he three times subjected to humiliating 'medical' examinations which had more to do with perverse sadomasochistic sex games than proper health care? Why does the German state still, now well into the twenty-first century, provide some people with 'special interests' such unlimited power over defenceless youngsters from the opposite sex?

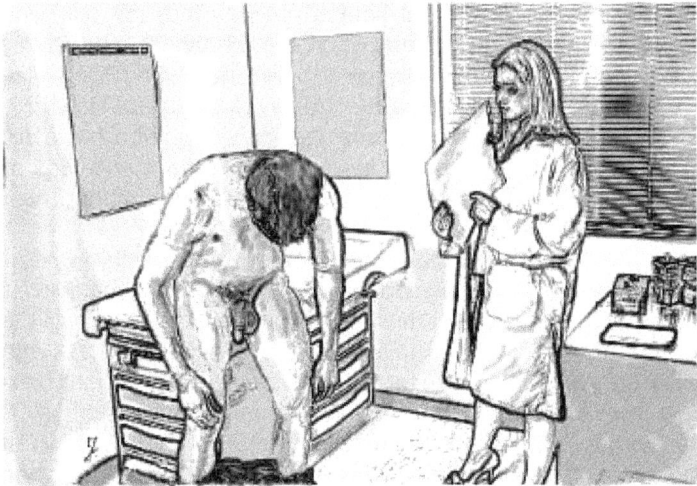

Looking for a Suitable *Musterung* Doctor

When these days - due to peaceful European conditions and a subsequently reduced need for conscripted soldiers - roughly every second young man is considered 'not suitable', these examinations have developed into little more than a state lotto. More than just ability nowadays will decide who has to serve and who not, a fact that provides the medical inspectors with more power than ever before.

Under such conditions it seems obvious that the one who 'behaves himself' will stand a better chance to be kindly exempted from duty and allowed to continue with his own life than the one who makes a fuss (and refuse to pull down his pants). If so, who would blame the individual who bows his neck, allows them to do to him what they want and tries to turn a blind eye to the humiliation - all in the hope of thereafter being allowed to leave the building as a free man?

Yes, this happens. Many young men, due to this understandable desire for freedom, will comply with whatever is asked of them. But, with this hope of a bonus at the end of the tunnel these individuals have also converted themselves into easy prey for their exploiters. In the long run that might be a very bad idea. All right, they *might* have achieved physical freedom for the time being, but, very often, what happened at the draft office made them prisoners of their past - and the term to serve for that negligence in protecting themselves could very well be life.

> The German Constitution Article 3: 1. All human beings are equal before the law. 2. Men and women are equal.

There will now be quite a few readers who would say: yes, of course it's bad when employees abuse their positions. It's horrible when it's about clerics, and it's horrible when it's about health staff. But, still, that's what can happen. At least, employers don't look for them. Not long ago I would have said the same. Until I read the following:

Medical Rape

Advert for Position by the Armed Forces

(This is NOT a perverted joke, author's comment)

For around one year Ms Dr X works as *musterung* doctor at the *Bundeswehr* draft office in Y-stadt. After ending her medical studies at the University of Essen, she looked for alternative areas of career and discovered the armed forces. The job as *musterung* doctor has turned out to be exactly as she expected it. Now the thirty-three-year-old's work day starts at 7.15 am with the first conscripts.
  'Of course it's embarrassing for them when the trousers have to be dropped. And there are so may rumours about these examinations. But, most young men take it all fairly relaxed. I have even experienced that some are happy that it's being done by a female and not a male.'

www.karriere.de/beruf/arbeiten-bei-der-bundeswehr-8315/5 - 67k - **Cached**

All right, what kind of job seeker is it who could possibly be attracted by an ad like the one above? To realise that fully we only need to swap the involved people's genders....
  Yes, this *is*, believe it or not, an authentic recruitment advertisement trying to attract medical doctors to the German armed forces and to its draft offices.... After two years research into this area of consistent, state-approved abuse I was still gobsmacked when I was presented with this ad. I could simply not believe it was true. Yes, what kind of person would be attracted to apply for a job?

Lars G Petersson

Employed as a Spectator

A good modern way of researching a sensitive area of interest is to have a look into internet forums. In there, protected by the virtual world's anonymity, people who otherwise would never dare talk openly about a difficult subject can do so. The issue around the *musterung* is here no exemption, and, thanks to that, I managed to get in touch (and also meet in person) with people who otherwise would have been beyond reach.

Anyhow, in the process of browsing this very special part of the internet, I was also in for a surprise. Not only annoyed victims and anxious teenagers but also staff - doctors and assistants from these specific institutions - took part in the discussions, or, when it came to the latter, I might rather say ridiculed those complaining. The arguments from their side would typically be generalisations like 'everything is being done according to the rules' and 'after all, this is how the law is and that has to be accepted'. On top of that, young people anxiously waiting for the upcoming humiliation were likely to be 'comforted' with statements like 'there is nothing to be ashamed of' and 'rest assured, we are used to looking at bums'.

However, for whatever reason, all of a sudden these voices died out. Orders from above? Looks likely. For me at least, it seems obvious that somebody from above had given clear instructions to stop staff-involvement in these internet discussions. Yes, almost from one day to another they were all gone. Nadine, Britt, Meike and all the others, they all vanished from sight. Suddenly there were no more comments like 'stop being childish' and 'this is a completely normal examination. What's the problem?' Suddenly the trivialising of young male embarrassment was gone. Suddenly it all just disappeared. Somebody must have seen these lady voices as a collective embarrassment for the institution...which they indeed were.

Be it as it may be with the reason for the lady commentators' collective retreat, before the ban I had secured one of these contributions as an example. Obviously, I don't know this woman's real identity, but, as I can rely on numerous other testimonies (also from insiders) I have no reason to distrust its authenticity. Therefore I will let this medical secretary who calls herself Helga represent the 'guild'.

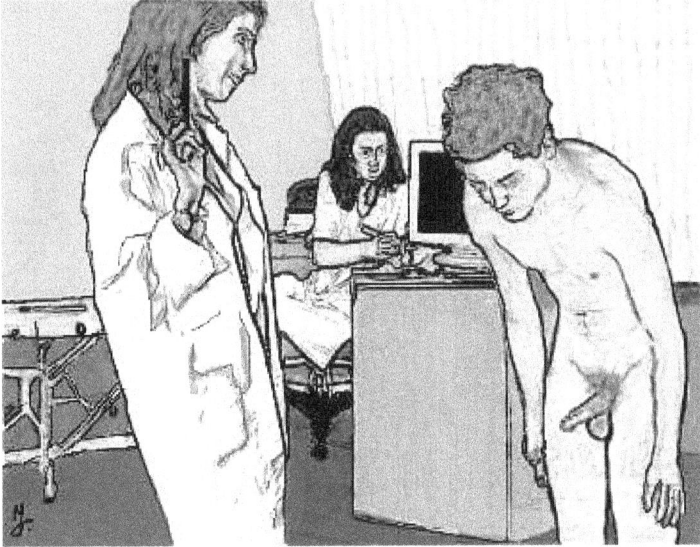

Helga is a woman who works in a *KWEA*, one of the sixty odd local institutions dealing with young people liable to the law of conscription. In this job she is, more than anything else, employed as a... viewer, spectator. Even if Helga never herself examines anybody, she still plays one of the main parts in the humiliation of young men. What is interesting here is the horrifying attitude and disregard for the mental suffering of other human beings that this letter portrays. As somebody who never has been forced to make herself completely free, Helga has made up her own firm position in the matter of mandatory striptease. What for Dieter and Sebastian has led to lifelong mental suffering is for her something 'completely normal'. At least that is what she says, and I am sure that this woman enjoys her profession; she seems to have no problems with what she is doing. At least that's how it sounds.

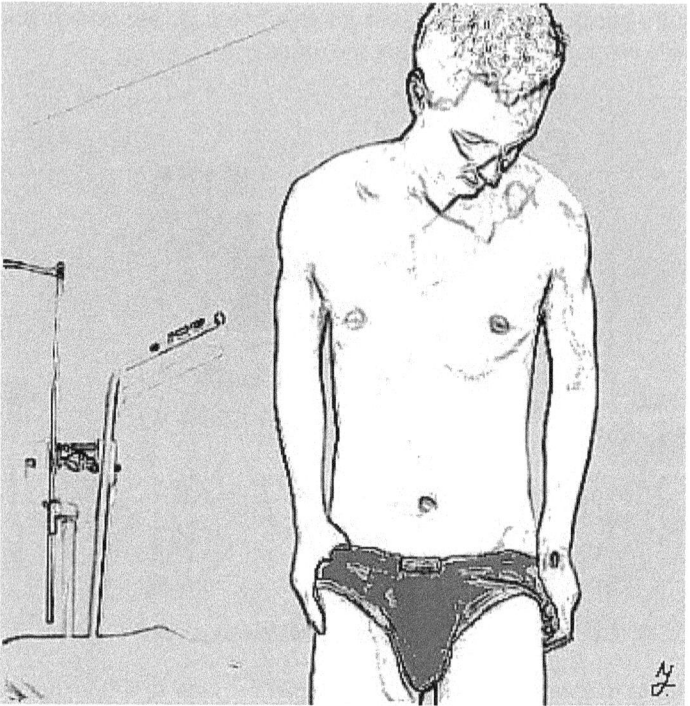

'Hallo, what can be humiliating about a medical examination? It is only about finding diseases and things like that. At our place it follows strict guide lines: after having identified himself, the young man is asked to get undressed down to the underpants, socks and shoes. That is nothing special; it's just like when doing sport and such activities. After that each person is called in individually. Assistant staff will then perform different tests and measurements: urine, hearing, sight, weight and height.

'Then the turn comes to the medical examination. At our place most doctors are women. Here the boy is first asked also to remove shoes and socks. One time one guy didn't quite understand. He asked: "only the socks?" Probably he knew from friends that he would have to remove everything. With a smile he was then told: "for a start only the socks."

'The examination thereafter follows strict guidelines and all findings are documented with numbers, so called 'Fehlerzif-

Medical Rape

fern' (numbers indicating 'faults'), which are dictated to the secretary as the procedure proceeds. Now everything will be examined: hands, nails, feet, mouth, jaws, skin, head and neck - just everything.

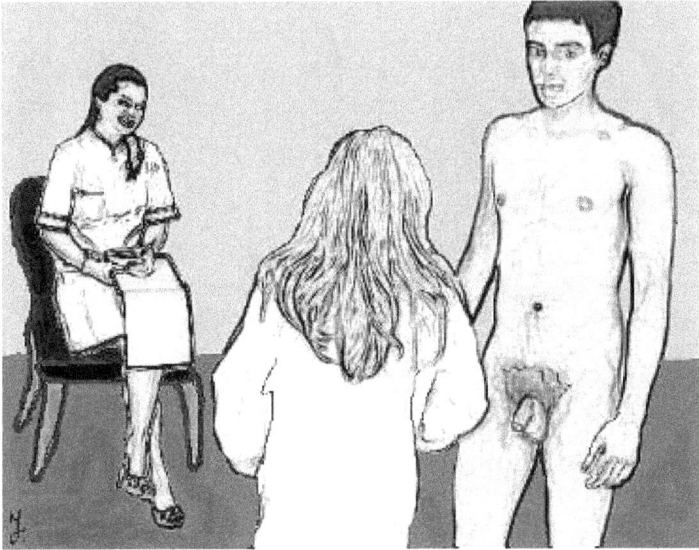

'The posture is checked, and the conscript is asked about his medical history, accidents etc. It's all strictly scientific and very thorough; nothing is left unnoticed. It is as by any doctor. After that has been done, heart, lungs and abdomen will be checked and the youngster is asked to do twenty squats before having his pulse and blood pressure measured.

'Then, at the end, comes what most guys fear: the genitals will be examined. Then I will hear: "remove the pants, please cough, pull back the foreskin, turn, bend forward" etc. I must admit, as a woman to watch a stark naked eighteen-years-old youngster pull back his foreskin can be quite exiting. As I after the training saw this whole scenario for the first time, I must admit it made me horny - especially because it was such a cute one. Yes, in this job one experience quite a lot.... Many times the doctor even pulls it back herself to check that it's all right. What precisely she examines there I'm not completely sure about.

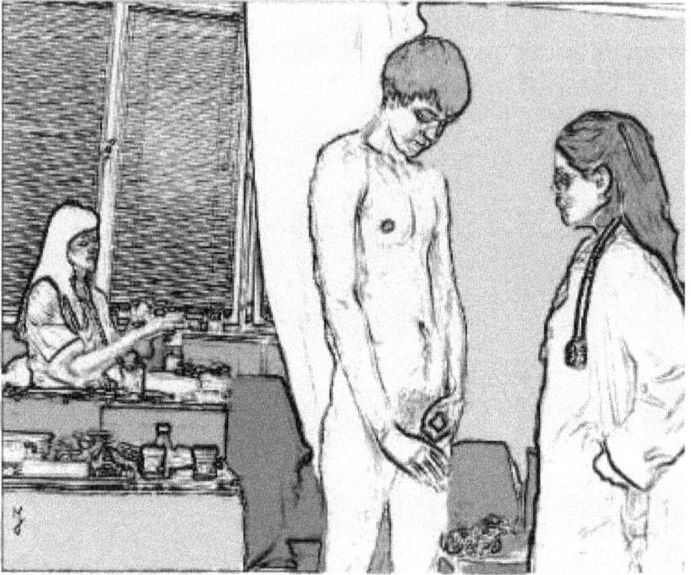

'After that the turn comes to the testicles, one by one, and finally the guy is asked to turn around, bend forward and spread his buttocks. At this stage, however, she just have a look but touches nothing. I cannot deny it's quite a funny feeling to watch a bent forward young man like that, to see his scrotum dangle there underneath his back passage. A *digital* examination of the anus, however, is only to be performed on those forty years of age and older. At our place I haven't seen that, as we are only dealing with young conscripts. After all that has been done the young man is allowed to pull back up his pants.

'When sometimes this "thing" shows it's alive, that can be quite hilarious to watch. Of course, for the boys such an event must be quite embarrassing, but, on the other hand, they must remember that it works and be proud of that. And one thing I can definitely confirm: it is definitely arousing to watch when a young man is asked to grab his little friend and present its "head".'

Secretary Ilse K.

Medical Rape

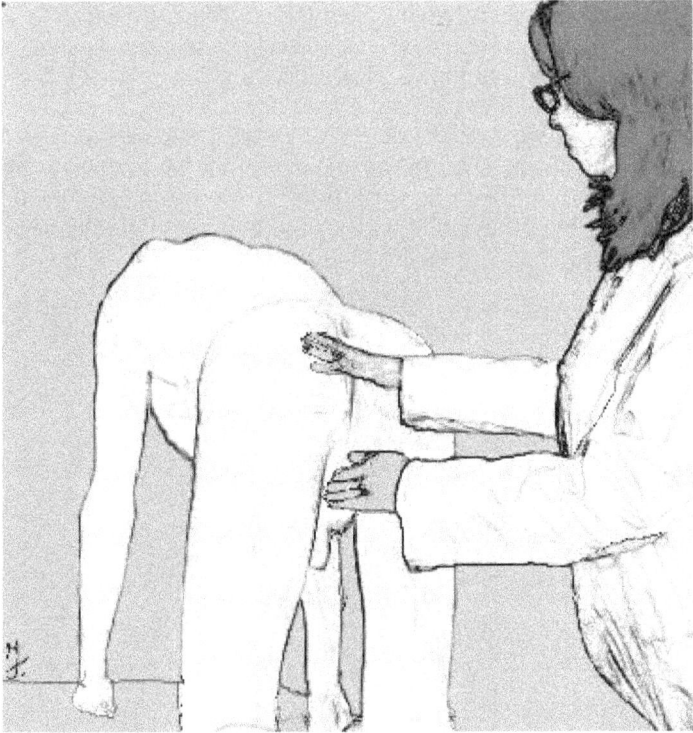

'Of course, a physical examination is mostly unpleasant. After all, who goes happily to the doctor? But humiliating? No, it is not. Of course, some young people are quite chocked as they are asked to remove their underpants. Sure, it might be unpleasant, but, after all, that's how life sometimes is, isn't it? No matter what, we have seen more penises, testicles and backsides than most others; so, nobody needs to feel he is anything special; nobody needs to feel ashamed. And, to be honest, that a young naked man, also with pulled back foreskin, can be an arousing sight for a woman, that is also something completely normal - nothing strange about that.

'At our place at least nobody has refused to strip and to show their parts. That would of course also be quite a childish behaviour. After all, this is how the law is: when they are eighteen they have to let themselves be examined, and then they of course also have to get undressed. If not, then the whole thing would be nothing but a joke. Wouldn't it also be a joke if something should be exempted from being examined, if penis, testicles and the anus should be a no-go-area? If so, why do it at all? What would be the point?

'In the end, no matter how you look at it, it's all positive: if one is not lucky enough, as most are, to be told they are healthy and sound, then he will be rewarded with being exempted from service. This way there is something positive in it for everybody.'

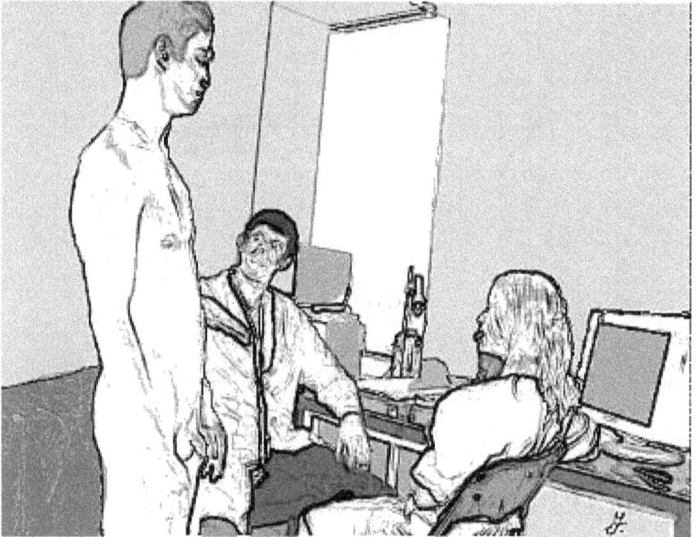

The situation in the draft offices, in the military medical departments and in the civilian institutions dealing with conscientious objectors is pervaded by a hierarchic relationship between the examiner and the person being examined. If he does not know his rights and stands up for them, he will be completely exposed to the whims and power of the doctor. Here it does not really help that he is never explained that he has a right to refuse or that he, like the female volunteer candidates, as alternative to the examination has a right to present a medical certificate from a civilian doctor of his own choice. And, just as little it helps that he is not told that he at least has a right *to ask* for a male doctor should he prefer that. Of course, having a right to ask does not necessarily mean much, as the large majority of these medical persons are female.... But still, not even to ask he is allowed.

Indeed, the situation for the young man is difficult. To be honest, he won't stand much of a chance. If the whole atmosphere is not enough to break his resistance other things will do. Most common would be threats of 'consequences'. For a young person this would be very difficult to withstand.

This far the talk has been mainly about the draft office. Even much more difficult it would be the day the same procedure is to take place in the barracks. A refusal here would be seen as disobedience and refusal to obey orders - a serious military offence. No, as we can see, there is not much help to expect for young people finding themselves in this situation, no matter if they are conscripted or have chosen to enlist.

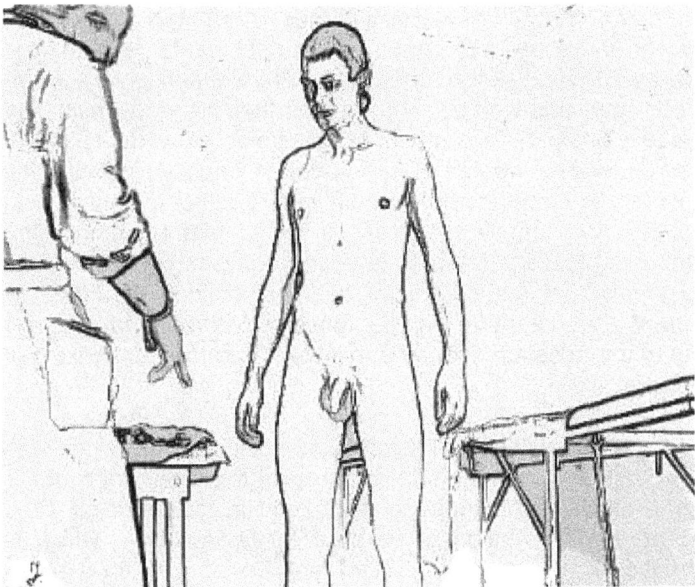

After all, so Are the Rules

Yes, Helga describes how things are. Everything is following a plan, and the instructions must be followed. No questions are to be asked; nothing is to be challenged. So it was, and so it stays.

But, there is an area where changes actually *are* welcome. Years ago the military was seen as nothing for women. From active soldiering they were of course excluded. Caring for the wounded was allowed, but, still, then it came to the other part of the military 'health service', *musterung* examinations, then it was again off limit.

In an old internal instruction, the *ZDV 46/1* from 1957, following was clearly stated: 'female persons are not allowed to be present when men are medically examined.' However, already at the end of the sixties these rules were 'forgotten' - though there seem to be no written documents declaring the change(!). The reason for that was the Equal Rights Act between man and woman. That means that this act, which was actually passed in order to bring into being *equal* rights, in this particular area worked in the complete opposite direction by creating extreme adverse inequality. From then on, supported by this law, female medical staff could perform humiliating strip examinations of conscripted (and enlisted) soldiers, while forgetting that the objects of their inspections would be all males, and that the reversed situation would be (and is) totally out of the question. Indeed a fairly perverted way of looking at equality.

Yes, for sure, the whole construction is sick. However, it is more than that: it is, as I see it, a clear breach of four decades of young German men's basic human rights, their rights not to be subjected to degrading and humiliating treatment (The European Convention of Human Rights, Article 3, which is legally binding, and the Universal Declaration of Human Rights, Article 1). According to the German Constitution, the state also has a duty to protect its citizens against such treatment. But, instead of doing so, when it comes to young men, then this same state has legitimised it all and hereby made itself into a lawbreaker. A reasonable high price to pay for giving some people 'equal' rights....

Medical Rape

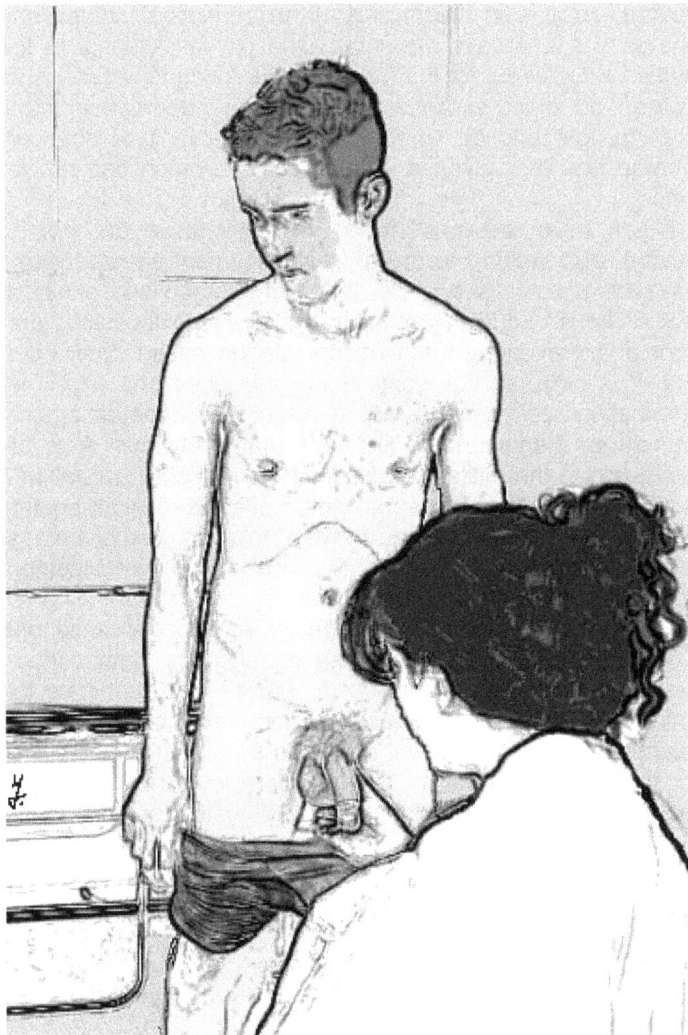

Do I need to say that I take equal rights seriously? In fact I do. With equal rights I mean... *equal rights.* Unfortunately, I am far from convinced that many others take it equally serious when they use the term. In fact, that seems to go even more so for the 'equal rights' institutions themselves and especially for those working there. So it is in the civilian world, and, of course, so it is in the military. With or without stripes and chevrons it is always the same, and I'm not kidding: in the bodies established for the purpose of working for equal rights in the work place exclusively women have democratic rights both to vote and be voted for. Yes, believe it or not, only women are here given a vote and only women can run for office....

If you have recovered from that, let's move on: yes, of course, also within the military establishment special bodies have been established in order to encourage and establish 'equal rights'. Sure, theoretically this is about abolishing present and preventing future discrimination based on gender. But, it is obvious, the whole thing only goes one way. Discrimination against men is not an issue: discrimination against women is. It shouldn't be like that; that is obvious. After all, according to the military forces' own equal rights legislation it is the clear duty of the equal rights officials to work against gender discrimination in all forms, including *sexual* harassment. And, there are no specifications in that announcement saying that this can only go one way.

So, let us go back to our specific topic: how could one expect anything less from these equal rights 'ombuds(wo)-men' than that they should put all efforts in to terminate the extreme sexual discrimination of men during the medical examinations? Of course, that should be an indisputable task for these officials. But, is it? No. There is nothing indicating that these women have done anything whatsoever to stop this abuse. Quite surprising, isn't it? After all, this group of people are extremely well informed when it comes to this subject, as a very large number of them are representing the medical services themselves.... So, are we actually talking about a conflict of interests? Are some of these equal rights officers actually in their daily work life part of the discrimination, part of the problem? Yes, very likely so.

No matter what, today, when it comes to 'equal rights' within the concept of the German military, then it is about positive discrimination for females, then it is about rights not duties, and, in the end, then it doesn't matter if innocent stripped young men are subjected to humiliating 'medical' scrutiny as a result of it all. That way, over the last four decades, the job of selecting young men for forced labour - whether in the military

Medical Rape

or in the civilian area as conscientious objectors - was taken over by volunteering women who, without ever having any legal duties themselves, with the Equal Rights Act as bizarre support, were given almost boundless rights not only to decide over the nearest future of young men but also to treat them as sub-humans.

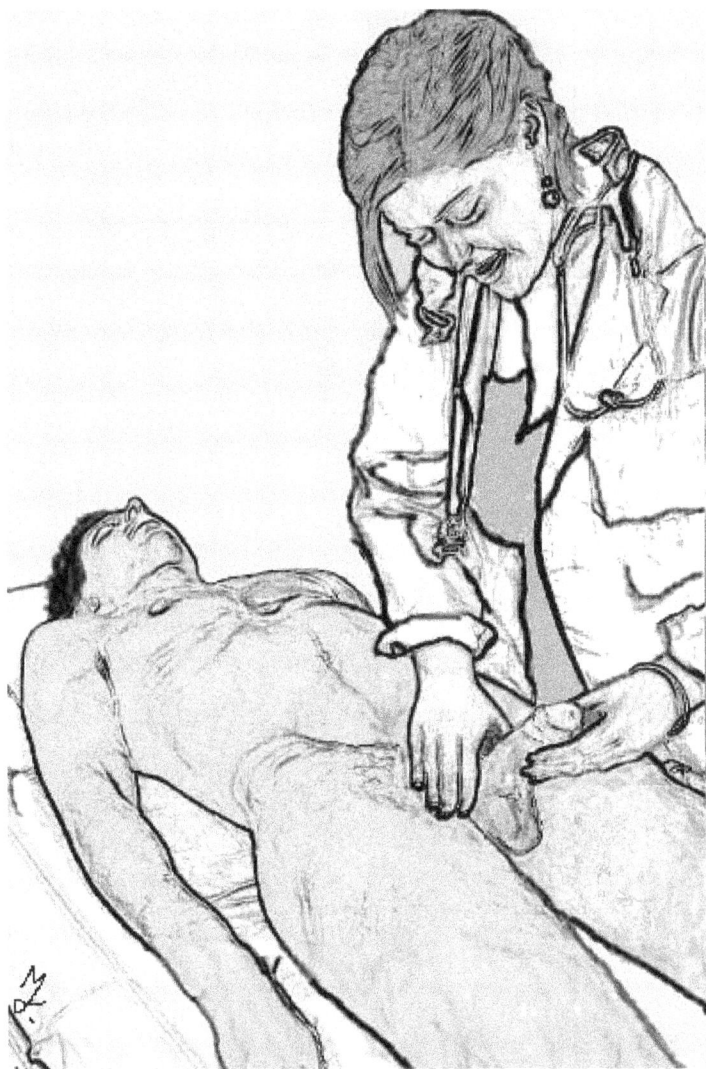

Lars G Petersson

Some people would call all this modern times.... 'Yes' to equal rights when that serves the purpose: 'no' when it doesn't. As a consequence of it all: today's *musterung* rituals must be seen as much worse for the victims than yesterday's strip-presentations among 'peers'. In those days at least they all had to go through it. That means, before getting where they had ended up, even the tormentors, the inspectors, had had to drop their pants and be thoroughly looked at. Yes, also those people had in the past been ordered to spread their buttocks for inspection. Contrary to most of their successors they knew how it felt like having to do so. Still, and that is another distressing side of this depressing story, it didn't keep them from doing it to others as soon as they were off the hook themselves.

> 'Next month I must attend *musterung*. I have just turned seventeen. Is it true that one has to strip stark naked. The thought about that frightens me. What would happen if my penis got stiff? That can happen in the most impossible situations. I am terrified. Can somebody help me?'
>
> David E.

58

Medical Rape

Some are More Equal than Others

So, how can it be that such conditions can be allowed? Isn't such horrendous treatment violating the Constitutional rights of the individuals and doesn't it constitute a serious breach of the Human Rights Act? Yes, how does the state and its authorities not only manage to defend compulsory military and civilian services in peace time but also the demeaning treatment that goes with it?

In fact, in politics and law making most anything can be exempted when and if it suits those who make the decisions. However, there is one important matter that cannot, and now we talk about what must be considered as the most absolute basic right for every citizen/resident in the country. For that constitutional right it is not in any way allowed to make exclusions. It is not allowed in any settings at all, not in schools, not in prisons or detention centres, and definitely not in the military - in fact nowhere. We are now talking about Article 1 of the German Constitution, the article that proclaims very clearly that 'the dignity of every human being is absolute and must not be violated. It has to be guarded and protected. It is the duty of the state to protect this dignity.'

It is in fact so that modern laws in many areas have impro-ved human conditions. And, believe it or not, this should not exclude soldiers and conscripts within the armed forces. Also these people are according to the law no longer allowed to be exposed to boot-camp drills meant to break down their personality. That's good, but, if it is like that, how can it then also be that the sexually degrading methods and rituals as we see by the forced examinations can be allowed to be carried on completely undisturbed by modern times? Is it because precisely that area, the shameless discrimination against males, is a massive taboo, something nobody would touch even with a barge pole, something that at any cost must be kept out of the public debate? It probably is, but we must also remember that the discriminating examinations are only the top of an iceberg; the most fundamental injustice is the law itself, the one that makes it all possible.

After all, only for them, for young men, is the law of conscrip-tion written. Reading that law feels like preparing oneself for not only 'doing time' but also for spending the next two decades on a kind of 'probation'. This is what it says: 'liable to military service are all male persons from the end of their seventeenth year of life who are Germans according to the constitution and who 1. have their permanent residence in the Federal Republic of Germany or, 2. have their permanent residence outside of the Federal Republic of Germany and either, a. had their previous permanent residence in the Federal Republic of Germany or b. are in position of a German passport or citizenship.'

Through this regulation the freedom of movement is automatically limited for this 'free' person. From now on he cannot go wherever he wants anymore: he might have to apply for permission. Very clearly the rules say that a male person after his seventeenth year of life has to apply for permission from the draft office if he intends to stay abroad longer than three months. The same goes for somebody who might have the intention to *remain* abroad after permitted time has expired. 'Permission for any such stay abroad can be given to a male person for the time he is not expected to be called up for service,' the 'free' young male person is 'kindly' told. Whether peace or war: this is the way freedom look like in a country that prides itself of being one of the freest in the world.

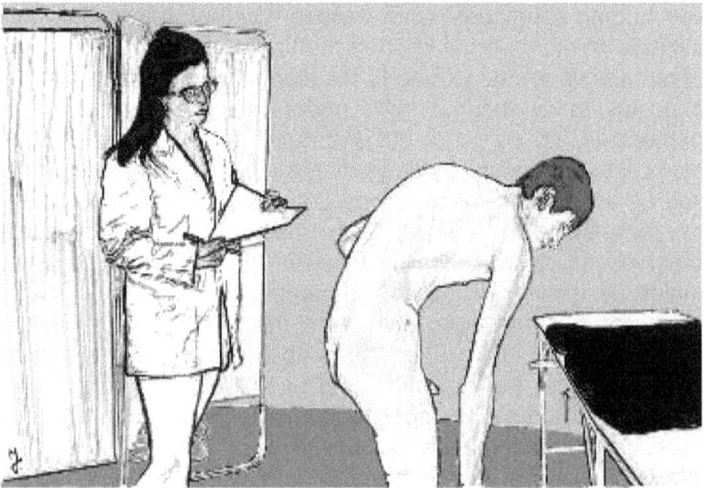

Medical Rape

Yes, it all starts at seventeen. From now on the young man belongs to the state and it all becomes serious. For example: if he does not follow the rules and turn up at the draft office when he is told to, he will be given a police escort to make it there. And, if making any further fuss, he could also go to jail. The Conscription Law, Article 3, says: 'national service means the duty to report, attend, present relevant documents and let one's body be examined for mental and physical ability to perform military service...' This examination is what they call the *'musterung'* and it is being performed in the various draft offices spread over the country, the so called *Kreiswehrersatzämtern.* (short *KWEA*). Everything that is going on there *should* be based on the following text: 'a person liable to military service is under duty to attend,' and 'thereby are such examinations to be carried out *which are necessary according to medical science to decide ability of the individual person to do military service.*'

'I don't know her name. Nobody introduced themselves. Without any "nonsense" the doctor just asked me to go behind the screen and get undressed. After I had stripped completely I was asked to walk back and forth in the room; she must have inspected my posture, I presume. After that she examined my back, before squatting in front of me and grabbing my testicles. When that was done I was told to turn, bend forward and spread my buttocks. For what must have been more than half a minute she then inspected my anus with a torch before she meant that everything was "OK".

'After that it was over to the bench to have pulse and blood pressure measured, then twenty squats and again pulse and blood pressure. Thereafter she waited for about a minute (what I felt like an hour) before she tested it again and asked if I was "nervous"....'

Wolfgang N.

Force that Must be 'Tolerated'

'Twenty long years I obviously could suppress the experiences from the *musterung*,' Dieter told me. 'But now I have to deal with the traumatic consequences of it all; I cannot push it away any longer. I constantly fight some sort of flashbacks, and I suffer from sleep disturbances and nightmares. Even if I am basically a very peaceful person I often experience rage attacks and can easily get irritated with most anything. Yes, I used to be a sensitive person who felt for others; today it feels like everything has changed: I no longer care, and that bothers me. Yes, the compassion I used to feel so strongly for other people is gone, has totally disappeared. Often I think about committing suicide. I don't want to live in this world any longer.'

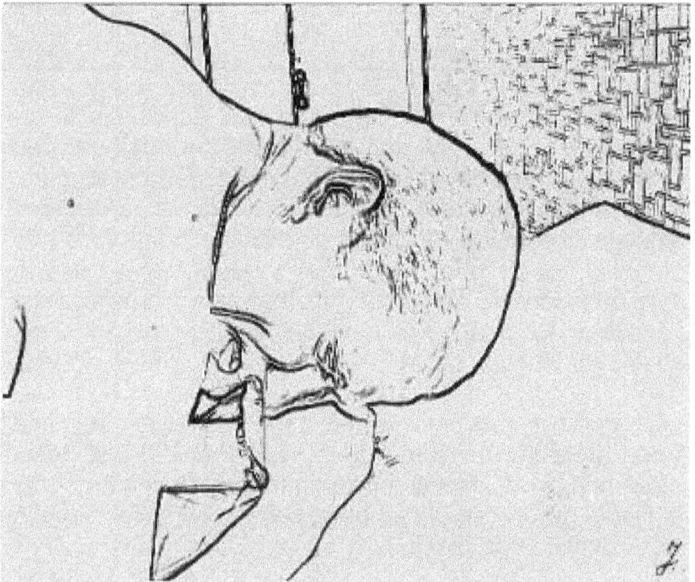

It all started with these humiliations. Dieter still struggles with the memories of having had to be checked and controlled from head to toe. He feels it was like a MOT, and he was the car - only a *thing*, not a human being. And, to be honest, he is right, nothing but that he was. Exactly as it is when the state

Medical Rape

orders a vehicle to be controlled it was for Dieter that day in April 1990 as he turned up for his *musterung* examination. Just like the auto mechanics would have had, also here the inspectors had their strict instructions to follow. Let's have a look at them.

According to the ZDv 46/1 (The Central Service Instructions) a full body medical examination is to be performed not only by the *musterung* but also at the beginning and end of both civilian and armed service. For men who have not yet served, this also applies if more than twenty-four months have passed since the last full body examination and/or if the findings by the first examination afterwards have been found to be incomplete.

This sounds indeed far more intrusive than ever needed and far above what the law itself actually decrees. Because, in the *legislation* around this area there is no reference to a *full* body examination. It is always stressed that it is entirely about *physical and mental ability for military service,* nothing but that.

However, let us disregard that fact and let us avoid going into details about all parts of the examination process which fall outside of the remit of this book; instead, let us concentrate on those specific parts of the body which if invaded by force or under pressure will affect the human soul most - even if they physically happen to be attached at the opposite end of the torso. Yes, contrary to what is legally required, the internal instructions - for whatever reason - do dictate that 'the male genitals and the anus are to be examined and inspected', and they do go on to tell the reader in detail about what he or she is to look out for.

For sure, this part of the entire examination process constitutes the absolute zenith of the victim's experience of being humiliated. But, there are other bits as well which do contribute in large mass to complete the picture of total submission. Of course, much of what now is to come is down to individual misbehaviour and abuse of power, but, there is no question, the central service instructions, the *ZDv*, are fundamental to it all.

One specific procedure that definitely would not need to be humiliating still ends up like one, not only because of the highly disrespectful way in which it is normally enacted but also because of *where* in the entire process it has been placed by the authors of the instructions.

In order to test the physical ability of the individual, the candidate shall, according to the instructions, be asked to perform twenty squats. To put it mildly, this is indeed a remarkably unprofessional way of deciding physical ability well into the twenty-first century.... But, worse than that is the extremely humiliating *manner* in which the process is to be carried out. And, shockingly true, it is all there in the instructions. First the half naked (in some cases already totally stripped) young man shall have his blood pressure and pulse measured. After that he shall be 'asked' to do twenty squats. Then, with one minute intervals, his pulse and blood pressure shall be measured until the level is back to 'normal'. Note, all this in presence of at least two (in most cases both female) staff.

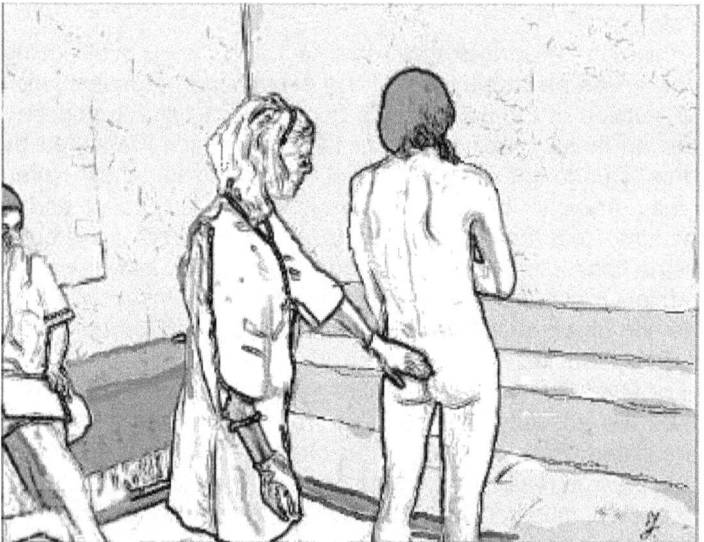

It should not be necessary to add the following to this story, but, let me do it anyway: most health care staff, at least those not working in German draft offices and military establishments, would know that it is fully normal for a patient in a medical consultation to present with a slightly higher blood pressure than that he/she would have outside of the consultation room, all this due to the stress of the situation - no matter if nice and friendly, no matter if being there by free will, no matter if fully dressed.

Yes, one of the most basic principles in medicine is not to rely solely on such measurements either for the diagnosis of high blood pressure or for the following up of the initiated treatment. Almost in all cases the person will be slightly anxious, and the result of a measurement during a medical consultation is therefore to be considered as unreliable. Research has shown very clearly that in the past many patients have been treated for high blood pressure without a definite diagnosis. They were just a bit nervous because of the situation....

Of course, all that was referring to normal civilian life. Let us now go back to where we came from and consider the disparity between the friendly atmosphere of such a consultation and the one of a military medical. Yes, that difference is enormous, and - I am sure anybody will under-stand - the individual's blood pressure will conform itself to that reality. To be honest, the doctor who would rely on such a measuring for a fitness certificate for war-duty must indeed have caused herself a serious insurmountable problem, at least if she ever one day would aspire to be taken seriously....

In light of what we here have talked about, the physiological 'examinations' at the draft offices at best can be called a joke or professional dilettantism. But, probably it would be more correct to call it a crime against defenceless young people, people who are unable to defend their human dignity against state legitimated perversion.

This far, when looking at the consequences of the official directives regulating this area, our focus has mainly been on the encouraged intrusions into the privacy of other people and on the instructions' advocacy of coerced, ethically repugnant, highly unprofessional and deeply humiliating gymnastic exer-cises in front of inspectors of the opposite sex. We will now look at other areas, some which hopefully will complete the picture. I am sure they will show the reader the full scope of this deep-rooted, state-sponsored disregard of other human beings' right to self determination when it comes to their own bodies.

No matter if we like it or not, everything that has been mentioned this far, the examined person, according to the regulations themselves, 'has to accept'. Consent from the 'patient' is not needed. This is the case no matter if he finds himself in a draft office, in one of the medical establishments within the armed forces or if he is dealt with by the civilian authorities handling conscientious objectors.

But, there are exemptions to that rule. Fortunately one would say. Medical examinations which could cause 'a considerable risk for the life and health of the individual' as well as surgery, also when the latter does not mean 'any considerable encroach into the person's right to physical integrity, are not allowed to be performed without the patient's consent'.

The following examinations are therefore only to be performed after the person has given his consent: lumbar punctures; sternal punctures; contrast examinations; isotope diagnostics; arthroscopies; biopsies of internal organs, and endoscopies of the gastrointestinal tract, the respiratory organ and the urinary tract.

'Had I just been a bit older, then I would have had another authority. But, at that time it was clear to me from the very beginning that I had to be subservient and do what I was told. My testicles were not *roughly* examined but in a very slow and thoroughly manner. She went from one to the other and back and back again. The foreskin was pulled back and forth three times by the lady. This far, it was the worst humiliation in my whole life.'

Lukas K.

If it wasn't as serious as it actually is one might even choose to consider the list quoted above as nothing more than an inappropriate bureaucratic attempt to be sort of funny. I mean it must be kind of a joke, mustn't it? How could one actually force somebody to such examinations? I mean practically, if someone really couldn't be 'persuaded'? For example, how would one by a forced endoscopy of the gastrointestinal tract actually pin down the victim/patient? How would one force him to co-operate and swallow? Probably quite difficult. Yes,

Medical Rape

also for the *Bundeswehr* this might prove to be a fairly difficult mission. Still, and this is what is important: that they this clearly write what exactly the individual *cannot* be forced to submit himself to makes it so much more clear to what he actually *can* be. In fact, what one cannot refuse to be exposed to seems to be all the rest - that means most anything....

So it is: what has to be accepted by soldiers - conscripts as well as enlisted personnel - are such medical examinations which, when carried out by professional medical staff, 'not with certainty or probability will lead to a worsening of the existing disease/condition, will not cause considerable pain and will not constitute a serious health risk.' For everything that can be included here the state and its armed forces also in the twenty-first century need no consent from the 'patient'. Of course, he belongs to the state; he has nothing to say.

However, should he still try to resist, he better think twice about that as well: 'culpable refusal to accept not unreasonable medical examinations (among them intimate examinations, author's comment) is an offence according to Paragraph 3 of the Law....'

With this background it is so much more difficult to understand that the office of the parliamentary ombudsman for armed forces personnel - which has a duty to protect the needs and rights of soldiers, enlisted or conscripted - had to spend three months before it was ready to answer a very uncomplicated letter regarding this matter. Did they really need to research that thoroughly something that must have been known for years? Or, was it rather so that the time was used in order to find a common language, a smart way out? Yes, probably they had spent the time looking for a secure legal way out of a very difficult position, a position they had brought themselves into by siding against precisely those people they had been put in place to protect. Tactically smart? Yes. Distasteful? Yes. Can it be forgiven? No.

Sorry for saying so, but this whole matter - that enforced medical examinations 'which are not combined with considerable pain or considerable risk to personal health' have to be accepted - reluctantly awakes in me some humble thoughts about a horrible but in fact not that distant epoch of medical history....

Lars G Petersson

Not only must the young man comply with everything that is asked of him at the *musterung* - also when it comes to scrutiny of his most private parts - but it will all continue and be repeated as soon as he is starting to serve - no matter if as a military conscript, as an enlisted soldier or as a conscientious objector. Also there this is part of the standard program, both when coming and going - and even in between.... True, the procedure is more or less always the same - as it must be done following an established form.

  This way everything is strictly following set rules - something that of course makes everything so much easier for the ones forcing themselves into other people's privacy. It frees the person from making up her/his own mind, or at least so they seem to reason. They, the doctors and their helpers, 'just follow orders' and are therefore free of personal responsibility. Or, are they really? Yes, at least they seem to think so. As they 'have to' follow the form and the instructions, how can it be the individual's responsibility when boundaries are stepped over, when human rights seem to be downtrodden in the process, when young people are caused permanent mental harm? Yes, how can it?

> 'At the second examination one year later there was only a male doctor present. To start with everything was all right. Then, however, he said: "I will now examine you rectally; please bend forward and relax." What I could just avoid at the first *musterung* examination I couldn't stop this time: as he put in his finger into my backside I got an erection. And, it would be worse than so: the doc then put in a tube, as he meant he had felt something that wasn't right. It hurt terribly, as the tube was thicker than his finger, but still I ejaculated. Thereafter I started to shake in my whole body, and I couldn't look the doc into his eyes. I was happy that no others were in the room....'
>
> Ulrich F.

This area of medicine never stops surprising me. For lumbar and sternal punctures, biopsies and endoscopies the consent of the patient of course is needed. Without that it cannot be conducted, as we earlier have learned. But, when it is about controlling the foreskin, when it's about checking whether or

Medical Rape

not that piece of skin can roll back and forth without problems, when it's about looking at someone's anus, then, all of a sudden, it's no longer - according to the authorities - necessary to ask for the 'patient's' consent....

After reading all this, is there anybody left who wouldn't see a sentence as 'the *musterung* process is free of charge' (which is written into the official regulations around this matter) as an unbelievably outrageous comment? A joke? Very unlikely. This comment can be read in the formal regulations, and is probably, believe it or not, meant as a generous favour, a sort of perk.

'After that I was asked to turn away from the secretary and pull down my underpants. Instead I pulled myself together and said: "I don't want to do that."

'"Oh, that's a very important part of the examination," she responded, and if I refused, I was told, it would be seen as an offence against the rules. I "would risk a fine". Threatened by that I bent my neck and did as I was told: I removed my last protection and stood stark naked in front of the two ladies. It was quite extraordinary. One of them, the doctor, sat on her chair in front of me and examined me "very thoroughly". I could feel how my blood went up in my head. Good, I thought afterwards, that it went that way and not the other.... How embarrassing if I had had an erection instead.... Thank God I didn't.

'"So, and then pull your foreskin back," she said. I was taken totally by surprise. What does she ask me to do? Still, I followed her orders.

'"And now turn around, spread your legs and bend forward." No, that was too much. I wouldn't do that.

'"No, I won't do that," I said.

'"All right, then you can get dressed and go. You will be called back."

'Today I know that it is all true what they say about these examinations. I have experienced it myself... and next year it will all be repeated.'

Andreas I

69

Lars G Petersson

Herzog Spoke to Deaf Ears

Also when it comes to the conscription law itself it does not seem like responsible politicians have taken much notice of a speech held in 1995 by Roman Herzog, at the time president of the Federal Republic of Germany.

At the celebration of forty years with the *Bundeswehr* - the 'replacement' of Hitler's 'defence' forces, the *Wehrmacht* - the president, lawyer and former member of the Supreme Court appealed to those in charge: 'the conscription is such a serious restriction to a young citizen's freedom that in a democratic state of justice this can only be justified when an external threat makes this unavoidable. In line with this the conscription is not a permanent unquestionable principle; it must always be dependent on the security needs of the state.'

Herzog went on to say that 'if we want to keep conscription, then it's important that we can explain why we still need it even if the immediate, external danger to the state has disappeared.' But, Herzog spoke to deaf ears. Nobody seemed to have listened to this man's words. As if preparing for the next war the armed forces fifteen years later still control and check as usual.

'As I was examined by the civilian authorities before starting my service as a conscientious objector the lady doctor asked me to pull back the foreskin. I was quite taken aback and surprised but did as she said. However, she wasn't completely happy with the result and repeated: "all way back". It was quite horrible to stand there in front of this fifty something woman and her young assistant. As she then finally had convinced herself that everything was alright with my foreskin, I was told to push it back out, turn around and spread my buttocks. When one day I am finished with the service I have been told it will all be repeated. I hope I can avoid that, but I don't know how.'
Lutz E.

70

Medical Rape

Equal Rights and the Constitution

The general instructions for the carrying out of medical examinations by the German military are the same no matter if the
objects are conscripts or professional soldiers. And, officially
the same rules and regulations should cover both men and
women. The same kind of examinations should be performed,
and, of course, in the same manner. After all, the emphasis is
on 'ability to serve and nothing else', isn't it?

Still, as we already have learned, there is a whole world of a
difference when it comes to these procedures - especially
when it comes to protection of the individual person's dignity
in the process of carrying it all out. Here, when it regards one
group, women, top priority is given to this protection, and
when it comes to the other it is totally disregarded, a complete
non issue. And, it is not just in *daily* life that this is obvious, it
is already there to read in the more specific and detailed
instructions which doctors have to follow.

Yes, according to these internal instructions men's genitals
are to be examined by inspection and palpation, but when it
comes to women history taking is considered enough. Only if
there is a specific concern, a gynaecological examination will
be considered - and then by a gynaecologist of the woman's
own choice. Interesting here is that also the anus is excluded
from inspection, again completely contrary to how men are
treated. Though there is no anatomical difference that should
prompt a different approach to the question of the need for an
inspection of this area, by women it is simply not done. Respect for the individual and the knowledge of this check's
uselessness comes here before the need to humiliate the
'patient'. That means that when it comes to women there is no
talk about military-style strip examinations in front of opposite-
sex inspectors - all in sharp contrast to what is forced upon
their male counterparts.

Yes, the differences are considerable. Male secretaries (soldiers working for the medical services) are of course completely excluded from examinations of women (even when it has
nothing to do with private parts or undressing) and male doctors are only used if nobody else is available.

The explanations for this gender-based discrimination are to
say the least astonishing. In one reply to my correspondence I

read the following: 'it is because the parts which need to be inspected and palpated by men are openly accessible. They can therefore without any problems be accessed and un-complicated examined....' With women, according to the same *official* view, 'instruments and special professional knowledge (sic) are needed,' and therefore these situations 'cannot be compared'....

Apart from the fact that this is an obvious breach of the constitutional right not to be humiliated and discriminated against, this statement also means that according to the Ministry of Defence no specific medical qualifications are nee-ded when attending to male genitals - because they are easy to see and touch.... This is indeed a remarkable point of view! To make it perfectly clear: this would be equivalent to a sce-nario where any basic trained medical should have the right to *force* upon any woman who attends his clinic (no matter why she is there) a check-up of her breasts, all this explained with the fact that they are easy to see and get access to....

> 'Last night I watched a *musterung* scene on television. It was exactly as I had experienced it myself. The young man had a nightmare; he hold on to his genitals and started to scream.'
>
> Aslan Y.

All in all, in the draft offices and related areas we find our-selves in the absolute epicentre of legitimate, discriminating treatment of men in Germany. Men liable for military service are here not only to be examined and evaluated for (forced) war (and civilian) service by women who themselves, due to their gender, are exempted, the same men are also (contrary to their volunteering officer-aspiring women 'colleagues') being subjects to extreme medical examinations where they, due to their woman inspectors' claim for 'equal rights at work', are forced to expose themselves to the most humiliating treat-ment, something which the other way around would be comp-letely out of question - all of this as a result of 'equal rights' going completely mad.

Precisely so, the respect offered women who volunteer to join the armed forces is on a completely different level than the one shown their male counter parts (*whether* conscripted *or* enlisted). As we already have seen, already from the start of their military career they enjoy a completely different protection of their privacy than what is offered to their 'colleagues'. First of all: out of deep respect for the female sense of shame the examinations of genitals are classified as damaging to the personal right of intimacy and therefore, as a rule, not performed. Would it be seen as necessary from a health point of view (what other reason should there be for such an examination?) to have a military woman's private parts examined, then that would be performed by a female doctor if ever possible.

In any case, the presence of *male* medical assistants (who still constitute the majority *within* the armed forces) in this connection would be completely and categorically ruled out; it would be totally out of the question. By no medical examination of a woman such a soldier would be present - completely regardless of the problem being looked at. Of course, all that has to be seen as an extreme contrast to what male conscripts and professional soldiers have to accept....

That leads me to the following: is it really so that the civil servants at the Ministry of Defence doubt that their own constructed concept of doctors' 'sex neutrality' can be extended also to embrace (their own) *male* doctors? In fact, it looks like that, and, if so, then this constitutes a very serious accusation against these employees.... Yes in fact, if so, then the authorities do not have trust in their own male doctors' ability to treat their female patients without resorting to unpermitted indecent acts. The question that then has to be asked is: why is nothing done about it?

On the other hand, if there would be no reason to assume that there should be a general problem in this field, then it would be of paramount interest to know why the otherwise hailed concept of 'equal rights' within the forces all of a sudden does not apply? Is it rather so that the gender indeed plays a very important part in all this? And, is it so that when it comes to the female *HUMAN* this is thoroughly acknowledged and respected, but, when it regards the male *THING* then one can forget all about it? Unfortunately, that's the way it looks.

One Has to Endure it All

For men liable for military service, duties and forced examinations do not end with completion of the basic service. For
many this is only the beginning, and, according to the law,
conscripts who already have served in the armed forces can,
if needed, again be called up for service. If that is the case,
then these young people will be ordered to subject themselves to renewed medical examinations (all included) 'if more
than two years have passed since leaving and/or if there are
reasons to believe that a change in their mental and physical
health can have taken place'.

In fact, at any time a person can be ordered to report to the
draft office and submit himself to new examinations. So it is
when a man is subject to what is called *Wehrüberwachung*,
the permanent state of being a reservist liable to serve
whenever requested. However, this duty is not reserved for
civilians. The same goes for professional soldiers.

During the time the person is subject to this *Wehrüberwachung* (for officers until age sixty, for commissioned officers age forty-five and for privates - as well as for men who,
for one reason or another, have not yet served - age thirty-
two) he has to arrange at any time that he can be contacted
without any delays, and if he is asked to present himself in
person, he has to do so immediately.

The restrictions to personal freedom go very far. For example: when somebody has served in the forces, the following
has to be accepted: on request he has to let himself be inocu-
lated to prevent infectious diseases (it is not his own choice);
if it is for him so decided, he has to accept medical interference even if that encroaches into his right to physical integrity
(that means, if they so decide, they can medically do most
anything they like with him); he must report without delay any
circumstances which would mean 'non permanent' inability to
serve for at least six months, and he must report without delay not only any new injury and disease but also any deterio-
ration in conditions he might have suffered from at the time of
the last medical. Finally he has to report without delay if he
completes a new professional education and/or training or if
he changes career to do something else. 'Big Brother' wants

to know everything about its possession. All changes have to be reported and it is always 'without delay'.

> According to § 17 of the Law of Conscription male persons have a duty to subject themselves to medical examinations. 'The conscript has to endure all examinations which are needed to decide whether he is able to serve (in the military forces).'

Also for under-age boys these are the rules to follow. As soon as they reach their eighteenth year of life (age seventeen) it starts, and from now on their basic freedom is restricted. 'After the seventeenth year of life male persons have to secure they can be reached without delays by the military authorities.'

From this point the affected can only enjoy restricted rights and does not have full freedom of movement. Important to stress: here we do not talk about people who have been found guilty of a crime; we talk about the innocent half of every new generation of citizens. Nevertheless, from this point every young man loses the 'firmly' in the constitution secured right of protection of his human dignity. For these people, those who now are at the beginning of their adult life, this protection is *restricted*.

No, even if they have done nothing wrong, even if they are not suspected of having committed any crime, they still are to serve time and they are still told to do whatever they are told. And, if they don't, others will see that they do. For example, if a young man does not present himself as he is told at the draft office he will be given 'police escort' to do so. And, if he does not show up at the barracks he will be assisted there as well. For that job the police can be given wide-reaching authority. In order to present the person at the draft office or take him to his place of service they are not only entitled to look for him in his accommodation or out in the public space. With exemption for night time they can also, if asked to do so and if they suspect he is hiding there, enter flats and houses belonging to other people. Also, still according to the law, cohabiting people have to accept that their flats are searched in order to look for the fugitive. There are, however, limits for what *these cohabiting people* can be exposed to. 'Non-permitted hardship against cohabitants must be avoided,' the instructions kindly say. But *'non-permitted* hard-ship' against the conscript must obviously not be avoided. Or?

Is this an unfortunate error, or what? Against the teenage conscript police obviously need not avoid *unapproved* of (i.e. *illegal)* force (i.e. *violence*)? Does the writer of this law (in reality: the parliament) actually accept none permitted (i.e. illegal) police force (i.e. violence)? It looks like they do. Unbelievable really.

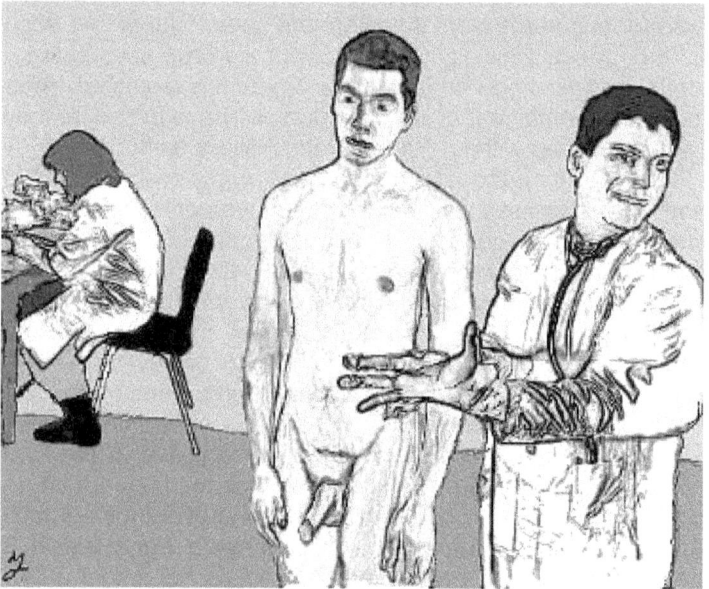

That such threats and limitations of freedom can be accepted in a country threatened by nobody is, to say the least, shocking - not least in light of the history of the country we talk about. But, we are not finished yet. Something will follow that has shocked me just as much. The basic rights of physical integrity (Article 2 of the Constitution), personal freedom (Article 2 of the Constitution), freedom of movement (Article 11 of the Constitution) and inviolability of the home (Article 13 of the Constitution), all those are, according to the law of conscription, to be limited. This law actually limits for these young people the most precious of all protective measures a state of justice has to offer its citizens, in fact precisely those which constitute the very core of the same state's right to define itself as such....

I find this nothing but a disgrace. On one hand the ruling body of the country expects the growing-up generation to develop into decent, law abiding, responsible citizens, and on the other hand the same body - in peace time, in absolutely no state emergency - removes from half of this young generation the most important rights which otherwise all individuals according to the constitution should be entitled to and which form the most basic foundation for a state of justice, equality and fairness. In fact, the safeguarding statures of the law on which the Federal Republic of Germany after the war was built has in reality never covered young men, and, well into the twenty-first century, they still don't.

'In a free county such abuse should not be allowed to take place. After all, the Nazis are history. Or aren't they? For the German armed forces and their helpers I have no respect. What about the constitution? What about the beautiful words in there about equal rights? What about those fine (empty) statements saying nobody shall be discriminated against because of their gender? In my personal sphere I feel they have seriously hurt me, and that will stay with me forever; I am pretty sure about that. Thanks to those responsible.'

Fabian Ü.

Growing up Among White Coats

Michael's constitutional rights were also at one point restricted. At the end these temporary restrictions became permanent, and his whole life stopped. At least, that is how he sees
it; it stopped before it had even started. In the end this man
never had to serve as a soldier, but the *Bundeswehr*, the
armed forces, still robbed him of most of what otherwise could
have become a 'normal' life.

  Michael's experiences with the military are now years back,
but still, in his mind they are his steady companions. The
memories are always there, as if it all was only yesterday.
Even if this man's underlying severe disease it the end 'freed'
him, he has never become a free man: the armed forces and
their medical friends still rule his day - today a quarter of a
century later. Yes, they are like old acquaintances, though
some he would rather do without.

'Already in the first year of my life I became ill with my lungs.
Therefore, growing up, I was always in close contact with doctors. It was all very difficult. Throughout my whole childhood
and adolescence I was frail, suffered from breathing problems
and was constantly on different drugs. Because of all this I
often missed out on school, and I had hardly any friends.

  'Then, shortly before I reached the conscription age, I was
started on a new drug, and an improvement in my condition
took place. Of course, that was good for my physical health
and well-being. However, it would have other consequences
as well. That I would soon find out, as I shortly after received
the first call from the draft office in Cologne. I was now nineteen years of age as I had to go for the *musterung*, my first
(out of three) military induction examination.

  'I didn't want to go there; I was anxious. And, I asked my
parents what they would do to me there. 'You will be examined,' was all they said. They probably didn't know much
more themselves, at least not my mother. Desperate I asked
my GP if he could give me a certificate about my condition.
"With that I might not even have to turn up, or?" Some documents he could give me, he said, but still, there was no way
out: I had to go. "Everybody must," I was told.

Medical Rape

'It was with a knot in my stomach I left for the conscription office. However, I was confident: "everything will be all right; of course, they cannot do anything but to declare me unable for service." At least I was convinced of that, even if at that time I didn't understand what the world '*musterung*' really meant. That would soon change, rest assured about that. It would soon be clear to me what it was all about....

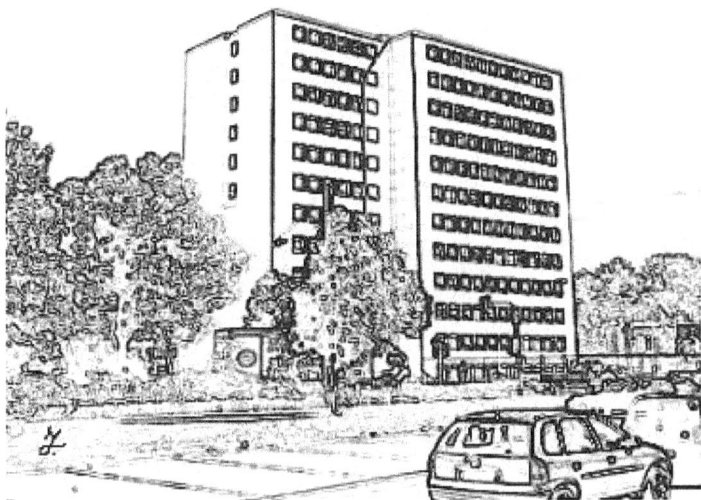

'On arrival I had to declare who I was; then I was told to strip down to trainers/shoes and swimming trunks or underpants. Not even a t-shirt was allowed to be kept on. That made it all quite frightening right from the start; I felt lost in there; it didn't make it easier that all the rooms at the premises seemed to be fairly big. In that half naked condition I would then have to walk around for the rest of the day - from one storey to another, visiting different stations in the process.

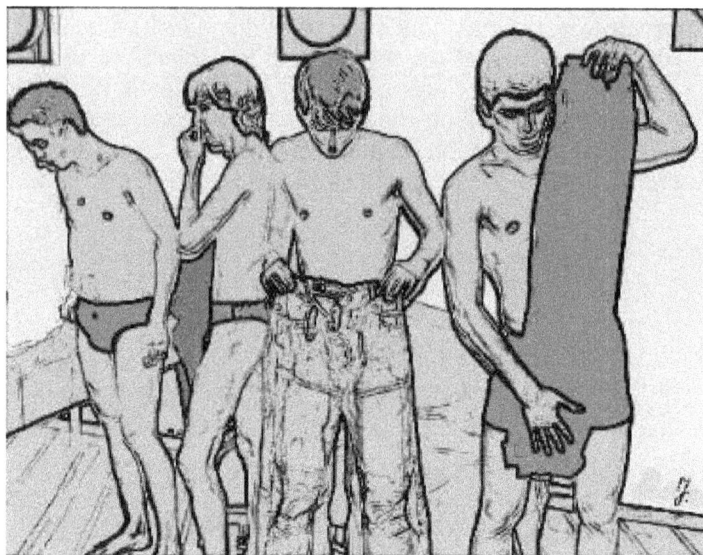

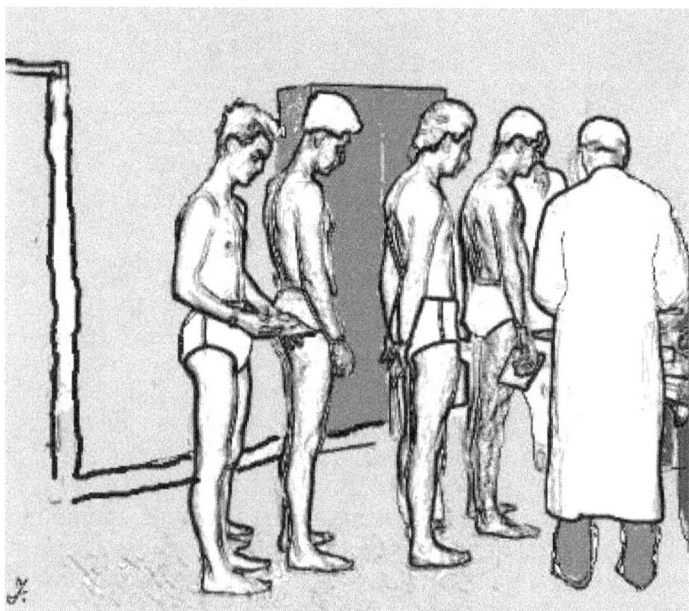

Medical Rape

'First of all we were sent down in the cellar for a urine sample - all youngsters at the same time. There was an older man down there who kept an eye on us. Of course it was unpleasant. Some escaped into the toilet cubicles which at least gave some protection; others, me included, had to wee in the 'pot' out there in the open. From this scenario I remember another boy who looked absolutely terrified.

'After that we were measured and weighed; blood tests were taken; hearing and eye sight were checked. And, of course, all the time we were dressed in underpants only. I haven't got a clue as to why. Sure, it was a very unpleasant experience. However, it would get worse: this was only the beginning. After all that had been completed, I was called to the main medical examination. I think it was up on the fourth floor; there I was asked to wait in a special waiting area until being called in.

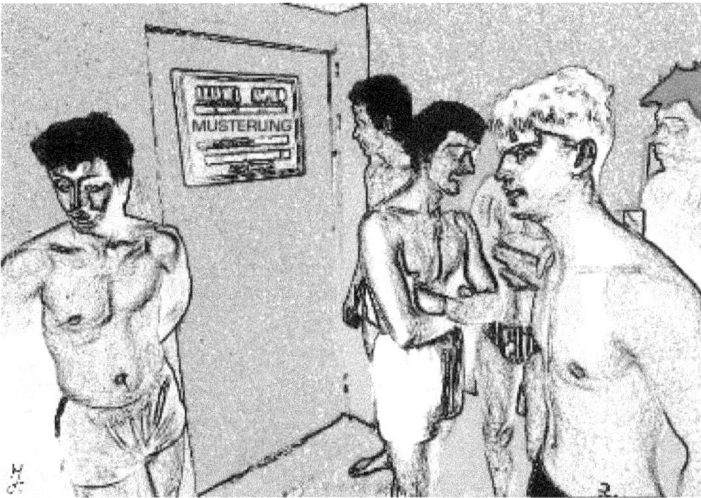

'After quite some time had passed, I was finally called into an examination room by a young dark-haired doctor. In there a young female assistant sat behind a desk. I was now in a fairly big room with large windows, and in the distance I could see the train station. I was told to sit down on a chair that was placed right in front of the woman's desk. That I didn't feel comfortable in that situation must be easy to understand. The doctor now started to ask me questions regarding my health story - all of it... including possible sexually transmitted diseases. That last question took me aback. I had never yet had a sexual contact at this time. What was I supposed to say? From where could I have had such a thing? It was all very embarrassing. I was very young, inexperienced - and half naked.

'To this examination I had brought documents about my asthma treatment. I thought that was important. However, this man didn't seem to pay much interest to them. Instead, he started to examine my mouth and teeth, and after that all the rest followed. I still remember every detail as if it had only been yesterday. My head and neck, my spine, everything was touched and inspected.

'I found this man extremely unpleasant; it was horrible to be touched by him. But what could I do? This young doctor and his female assistant could obviously do whatever they wanted to me. On top of it all it appears as if they had saved their best bit for the end. Precisely so, as I at the end of the session started to believe that there was nothing more to come, I was, to put it mildly, in for a shock. Yes, I had been too quick to celebrate.

'The doctor now stepped to the left and indicated for me to follow him. I had no idea as to what to expect. There was a square marked on the floor and right there I had to stand, I was told. In this position I was about two meter from the wall on which there was something I was unable to identify. Still today I ask myself why I had to stand right there on this marked space. Were they taking a photo of me? If so, why? I will most likely never find out.

'Right behind me the assistant was sitting, and I felt her eyes on me. Then the order came: "pants down to the knees." I had learned to obey people in white coats and did what I was told. I now stood there stark naked in this big room, and it felt like it was getting ever bigger and I ever smaller. I knew the woman sat behind me; I knew she could see everything that was taking place. But this was only the beginning; it would get worse: I started to get an erection, and the doctor starred at it. I felt ashamed.

'The man in white then stepped up right in front of me, and now he had his gloves on. Standing there like that with no-

Medical Rape

thing on, I felt totally humiliated and scared shitless. I could just as well have been standing on the market place encircled by people. I was defenceless. I could do nothing to protect myself. He now checked my testicles, moved the penis to the right and to the left and touched the tip of it. After that he dictated a number 'two' to his secretary, pulled of his gloves, throw them in the bucket and walked a few steps to the right over to the desk. I followed him with my eyes. He looked back at me, and I looked at him questioning. First at this point he indicated that I could pull my pants back up.

'I feel extremely humiliated by this horrible experience. I was shocked at the time, and I am still embarrassed by the memories of it. I am extremely angry with the doctor and his assistant. How *could* they do that to me? And what had been the purpose with the marked area on the floor where I had been asked to stand with my pants down? Did they take a photograph of me there?

'At the time I was devastated with shame, but more was to come, as I, despite my poor health and significant medical history, was not found permanently unable for military service, only temporarily. That means I would have to come back..... Today all these years later I am so angry with myself for not having had the courage at the time to refuse being treated like that. Why did I let them do that to me? Why did I allow them to ruin my life? Of course, the reason was simple: I was just so young and so inexperienced. For them I was easy prey; they could do what they wanted to me, and that they did.

> 'What I think was the worst was that I knew from before, from friends, what I had to expect in there. I thought all the time at what would come at the end and was terrified by the thought of getting an erection.'
>
> Christian A.

'After this first *musterung* I again suffered numerous attacks of serious breathing problems, probably exacerbated by the trauma I had been exposed to. After all, there is a psychological aspect to asthma as well, and it could have done me no good that my life from this day was totally dominated by fear of soon having to go back - to have to taste more of the same.

'This waiting lasted a year. Then the letter arrived, calling me back for another assessment, this time at the draft office in Bonn. At this place everything was sort of smaller, but the feeling was the same. To start with it was all a repeat of what had taken place the year before. But soon I was to realise that there was at least one change in the procedure: this time it was not a male doctor who would perform the examination but *two* women. Apart from that and the initial stuff, that's everything I can remember from then on.... Apart from that everything is gone.... Nothing else I can recollect, absolutely nothing. There must be something that blocks it. I have thought a lot about this in recent years. What was it that was so terrible for me that day that my mind in order to protect me has banned it from my consciousness? I have no idea. I can only suspect. Anyway, one thing I do know: once again I was declared unable 'for the time being' and 'would be called back later' for one more evaluation.

'In the time between this second *musterung* and the third, my breathing problems were getting ever worse. They were now extremely difficult to control. I was, to say the least, in a desperate situation: I suffered frequent asthma attacks... and my mind was totally absorbed by the fear of the next strip examination at the draft office.

'When the call then again came I brought with me a recent x-ray and left home with only two thoughts in my head: that I this time *had to* be exempted from service and that I would again have to stand there stark naked. All right, let me now go directly to the main medical. The doctor was a woman around forty years of age. She was extremely thorough. The examination took place in a smaller room, and an assistant who took notes was also present. This person sat close to the door and had the whole room in her view. First I was told to remove socks and shoes and position myself, still dressed in shorts, on a couch for the first part of the examination.

'Thereafter I was asked to do squats. While trying to do that, I slightly hit the desk and almost lost my balance. The lady obviously found that amusing, laughed and pulled me over to another spot. However, I didn't find the situation as hilarious as she obviously did: I was too ashamed. After all, I was a grown up man, twenty-one years of age, and here I was treated as a little boy. It felt like I had to do all these gymnastics just to entertain these ladies.

'After I had done my twenty squats I was told to sit down. The doctor counted my pulse and announced: '200'.

"'That's too much!"

"'I'm nervous," I exclaimed, and, to be completely honest, that was more of an understatement than exaggeration. By telling her, I sort of appealed to the lady to spare me more of the degrading part. Yes, this time I knew perfectly well what was in store for me: soon I would have to strip totally in front of these two women. I knew that, and, to be honest, I hadn't much hope that any appeal would make much of a difference. She seemed like someone who enjoyed dominating me; of course she wouldn't miss out on some fun.

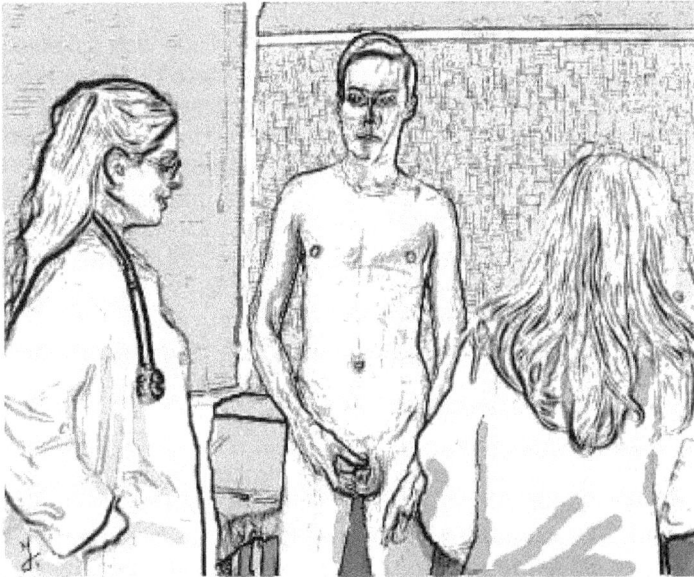

'Then the moment had arrived. "Remove your pants," the woman told me. As before, I had no courage to say no; I had no courage to refuse. And, apart from the shame I felt, I only had one more thought in my head: I wanted desperately to be found unfit for service. In order not to jeopardize that, I would probably have done most anything to satisfy the examiners.

Yes, they had complete power over me. I was totally in their hands.

'Obviously in order to check my gait, I was then asked to walk back and forth a few times across the floor. After that, with me placed right in the middle of the room, totally without protection, she went straight to my bollocks.

'"Please, pull your foreskin back," I was told to my horror. I did so, but obviously not good enough. "Further back, please!" I continued to follow her orders; what else could I do? It was all quite odd really: this was practically my first "sexual" contact with a woman (as I don't remember my second *musterung* examination…), but I had definitely expected it to be different.... As I at this point still had the words of the family GP in my head - "they will not take him" - I just tried to endure all the humiliation in the hope they would at last let me have my freedom.

'Finally I was allowed to pull on my shorts and was asked to follow another lady into the next room. In there I had to stand in front of a group of doctors. It was extremely difficult, as I was encircled by all these doctors, three men and one woman - the same woman as before. It was like some kind of interrogation regarding my health: my body was inspected from all sides. I had the feeling that I was totally in their hands.

'On top of that there was an assistant present as well, and I remember another lady who came in with all documents. The lady doctor then left for a short while, and during that time one of the others read in my papers and in the medical cert I had brought with me. The other two discussed between themselves. Myself I was standing there on the spot I had been shown and felt as if I was in court.

'Then "my" examiner came back in through the door with the x-ray pictures in her hand. I felt such hate towards her in that moment. I thought: if I really was to become a soldier, if it really would come to a war, if our country would be attacked by enemies, should I then have to protect a person like her? Would she then be what they so often call one of the "innocent civilians"? And, would I have to be one of the (automatically "guilty") soldiers who would be asked to sacrifice my life in order to save hers? Could my country really expect all that of me? Could my state genuinely expect me to make such a

Medical Rape

sacrifice for a person who had treated me in such a nasty and disrespectful way?

'As far as we can see your lungs are all right,' I suddenly heard her saying, as I woke up from my day dream. Obviously, if the lady doctor had ever been able to, she would have commanded me off to war service. To me she was such a cruel woman. Would she really have been like that if she also had seen me at home struggling to breathe? Would she then still have seen me as ready-for-use cannon fodder? I was angry at this woman; I was angry at all the others as well, and still I am.

'One of the doctors then asked - he appeared to me as the friendliest of them - whether I was in treatment for my allergy. The question took me by surprise. Had they not read the papers? All right, I then told him that I was on weekly injections, and that information (which of course was there to read in all my medical certificates) then finally - after all these 'examinations' - turned the case in my favour. Of course, the lady doctor was clearly unsatisfied with the turn of the case, but to the others it was now obvious that this condition could impossibly be combined with a life in the army.

Yes, so it happened that I, all of a sudden, was let off the hook - at least for the moment. Correct, entirely free I wasn't: if my health would ever improve they would call me back for another evaluation.... Yes, I was too ill for the moment, but, of course, that could change. If future treatment was "too successful" they would come back for me.

'I left the building as quickly as I could, and, as I reached the street, I breathed the air of freedom. It was like if I had been set free from a prison. From now on I tried to forget all about the military. However, that was difficult. For years to come I just couldn't get it out of my mind that they at any time could just call me back for new examinations - just to see if anything had changed, "for the better". Today I find all that extremely cruel as I from that point in life had to live in a constant state of fear and anxiety that another letter would arrive in the post.

'Not before I finally turned thirty-two (the legal upper limit for calling up a new recruit) I became a completely "free" man. First after reaching that age I so to speak was allowed to be in good health, free of symptoms. Forgive me for saying this, but, I *am* bitter. Had these "professionals" ever taken my medical history seriously they wouldn't have had to call me at all. I was totally unable for any kind of military service; my lung capacity was nowhere close to what would be expected. Still, three times they had to check me, and three times I had to show them my genitals. I still believe they were much more interested in those parts than in my serious breathing problems. This way these people ruined my life. They had total power over me, and they seemed to enjoy it. What they did to me back then now follows me from early morning till late evening. I cannot get it out of my head. Still this day after so many years I have a feeling that my body belongs to somebody else; it's not mine: it's theirs. That is probably how they wanted it.'

'The experience has burnt itself into my brain. With me is a constant image: I see myself with pulled down pants in front of the doctor in Dortmund - and behind me the assistant watching…. I still feel she is looking at me.

'I actually would like to meet this woman again; I would like to tell her how I felt that day and how it all has stayed with me. Whether or not she has ever made herself some thoughts about how her very presence can have damaged me (and all the other young men) I don't know. I presume she hasn't. For her it was probably just a job, just as it was for the lady doctor. In all likelihood they both just "did their duty"….

'The people who dealt with the Jews in the concentration camps, stripped them of their clothes and forced them into the "showers", they also just did their duty, didn't they? Just as the men who as soldiers raped the enemies' wives did theirs? Executioners also just do their duty, don't they? Yes, so it goes, on and on. What kind of world is this?

'The *musterung* is indeed a strange thing, a perfect tool with which the state makes young men feel hate. I am no longer a young man, but since the induction examination I hate this state and the people behind it.'

Sascha O.

Medical Rape

Childhood and Adolescence

For Michael it all began much earlier in life. As he was only one year old he was taken ill with his lungs, and it got worse as the years went by. 'I could hardly breathe when I tried to play with the other children on the play ground. Maybe it was because I was ill and frail that I also was bullied throughout school. Due to all that I stayed at home as much as I could and had practically no friends. After all, who wants to have a friend who is always ill? So it was: at home I often sat resting my head on my supporting arms - as breathing when laying down often was very difficult. I also had regular asthma attacks in those years.

> 'Three times they called me to *musterung*. The third time there were two women there and they told me: "you have too small testicles; you have to be seen by a urologist and be thoroughly checked."
>
> 'Off I went to the consultant whose only words were: "this doctor must have no idea about what she talks about. These testicles are just normal; there is nothing wrong with them."'
>
> Werner D.

'As my health didn't improve just the slightest bit I was sent to a health spa. The air there was of course better than it was back home. But, the effect wasn't long lasting: as soon as I was back home the asthma attacks were back as well - now even worse and more frequent than before.

'On top of that, the completely different conditions at the health resort had given me quite a shock. In fact, it was at this time in life I had my first taste of what would later become my ordeal.

'Before every stay in these health centres I was to be exami-ned at the *Gesundheitsamt* (the civilian health authorities which also perform medicals on conscientious objectors, author's comment). Being examined there meant having to strip of all clothes. I had to do that in presence of not only the doctor but also my own dad. That I found extremely difficult. After all, in our home nakedness was taboo and never prac-tised in front of others.

89

'In the spa, however, just as in the *Gesundheitsamt*, they took no notice of such "weird habits". Yes, it was the same there: "forget any privacy needs you might have as soon as you can". Already after the first time in this health resort (age seven) I tried to avoid ever going back. But, unfortunately, I was too little to make my point and be heard. So, before finally getting my way, I had to experience it all one more time. That was two years later, and I was nine.

> 'What can someone like me do against the omnipotent state? Absolutely nothing. Therefore, for a very long time I have seriously thought about committing suicide. Only when I am dead I can be free.'
>
> Mario B.

'At the arrival in these places all children (genders divided) had to undress completely and thereafter wait in a long row for the medical examination. For us boys this was even worse, as all staff were female.

'During my second stay we went once a week to a swimming pool. All swimming trunks were kept in a box in the home. One time my trunks were missing, and, to my horror, one of the women just told me to go without.... As I was the only child without swimming trunks in the pool it was a terrifying experience for me. After all, I was only nine years old and away from home. Of course I run as quickly as I could as soon as I was allowed back to the dressing room. For the next day at the pool my trunks had to my relief been found.

'Once a week we had to have our temperatures measured. The procedure was as follows: one of the staff entered the dormitory; we were asked to remove our pants and place ourselves on our stomachs in the beds; after that the woman put a thermometer in each of our backsides. Like that we had to stay until she came back to check our temperatures. I felt embarrassed by it all. I have never understood why it had to be like that. This embarrassment I at least think they could have spared us. After all, we were sick children who needed care.

'Also in the evening we had to strip completely before we were allowed to put on our pyjamas suits. Underwear was not allowed. As I was used to something else back home I once

Medical Rape

tried to put on underpants after I was already in bed. I managed, but the bed made noise and one of the staff came in.
She demanded to be told who had made such a noise, and
the other boys then pointed at me. As punishment I was told
to leave the room and sit outside on the staircase. I did so
and started to cry. The woman then obviously felt sorry for
me, and I was allowed back in.'

So years passed and at the age of eighteen Michael received
the call from the draft office in Cologne. It was a fairly unfriendly letter. From a state body he had never before received anything and today he says: 'I was shocked by the style.
If I failed to turn up I could expect to be taken there by the
police, it said; there were even threats of being arrested and
sent to prison. I wouldn't risk that: at age nineteen I went for
my first *musterung* examination.'

'As I was *mustered,* there were three women (one doctor
and two assistants) present as I stark naked had to make
squats and spread my buttocks. On top of that I had to pull
back my foreskin and the doc grabbed my testicles.'
Udo C.

91

Lars G Petersson

Already in Childhood it Starts

Three *musterung* later and Michael's life was ruined. To me it's obvious: this man is a victim of a fairly German obsession not only with nakedness but also with medical checks and controls - needed or not, wanted or not.

Today, in civilian life, medical examinations are (generally) performed with (hopefully) more respect for the individual patient's privacy than was the case before. However, that wasn't always the highest of priorities in the medical field, and, at least when it is about people under some kind of duress or dependence there is for sure still a massive problem in this area. Especially children, defenceless as they are by nature, are easy prey for abusive therapists - just as they are for preying clerics, as we have seen evidence of in recent time.

I will not try to kick start any competition about who is worst; I only want to stress that it's evident that also the healing professions have their own black sheep; the Catholic Church has no monopoly on that. I have no numbers; I cannot have any, but traumatic experiences due to abusive behaviour by medical staff and their assistants are common and regularly reported. Also here, children are very often the victims. This way, for many of those with painful memories from military examinations, these might 'only' have been the straws which broke the camel's back. The whole aspect of humiliating medical examinations can very well have started many years before. In fact, the first experiences can go all the way back to early childhood.

Especially with boys very little care has been shown for their right to privacy and protection of their dignity when going to the doctor. For example, at school examinations in Germany in the fifties, sixties and early seventies young boys were often completely denied any safeguarding of their modesty. Common in those days were obligatory nakedness by medical examinations and this often in presence of females - even those who had nothing whatsoever to do with the procedure itself. In the worst cases reported even same-age girls could be present (of course fully dressed) - something which reversed roles would have been completely impossible. If we want to, we can choose to see all that as an early preparation for what was to come....

Let us have a closer look at this. Let us ask somebody who knows. What about a former child? After all, we were all once one, though some people might have forgotten. 'As a child I always had to undress completely, and then penis and testicles were examined. Sometimes it even hurt physically. I had no idea as to why it had to be like that. Nobody told me what it was for.'

Another writes like this: I came into the examination room and in there were already two of my class mates. Both had stiff penises, and now also I was told to strip down to the socks. After weight and length 'the rest' followed. As she was at the penis she declared my foreskin to be too tight and, without asking me for my consent, just forced it up. All that right there in front of my friends.... Super embarrassing it was. I was really angry with the doctors in those days. What a bunch of pervies!

One ninth-grade boy describes his memories like this: 'all the boys in my class were told to go to a specific classroom and in there to strip to the underpants. After that we were measured and weighted by an assistant; she also did sight test on us and so on. Then we were taken into another room to be examined by the doctor. In this room there were always two or three boys at the same time - one who was being examined, one who was on his way in, and one who was about to leave. To my horror, also our teacher was present. She sat beside the doctor and could see and hear everything that was being done. At this examination we were completely naked. The doctor had a look at my anus, and at the front he examined very thoroughly.... As probably most of us, also I got an erection.'

Of course, in all these cases we must recognise that this was sexual abuse. How else can it be classified? No, that's the word, and, what makes it even worse is that it was all committed by people employed to *protect* children.... There should be no need to stress: such appalling behaviour on behalf of teachers and doctors is extremely bad for the growing up child, and, what we must never forget, it prepares for a submissive adulthood. The one who has got himself used to such medical examinations as a child is very likely not to defend himself against continued abuse even after reaching maturity. This way the uniformed school doctor transforms herself into the uniformed *musterung* doctor and the now grown up boy continues to let them do what they want to him. He has forgotten to protect his own body. Or, should we rather say, he has never learned to protect it against preying adults. This is actually something extremely serious; the school took its duty to prepare its students for real life a little bit too literal....

How deep mental disturbances due to such treatment of young people go, and how widespread it was and is, that is of course impossible to say, not least because this subject is a major taboo. Also here the victims stay silent and nobody will admit they were deeply hurt. Only in recent years it is recognised that also young boys can be victims of sexual offences and not just by men but also by women. I think it's time to put an end to it.

> 'Right now my mental state is calmer, maybe because the suppression works better than before. I am less depressed and there are no nightmares. Hopefully it stays like that. I don't want to spend my whole life with these thoughts; I don't want to have my whole life ruined.'
>
> Dirk V.

Very often these days the talk is about sexual abuse of children and young people. It is not a pleasant 'new' topic to discuss, but, unfortunately, whether we want it or not, it was a factual part of the past, and, even more unfortunately, it is a factual part of today. Therefore, we must realise that this kind of human behaviour was and is more widespread than we have ever expected, and we *must* do something about it.

Yes, again and again we read and hear about it in the media. Sometimes children's homes are under scrutiny and, on other occasions, adults preying on the internet are getting the attention. In recent time, however, the focus has mainly been on the abuse within the frame-work of the Catholic Church. Conclusion: it is most everywhere to be found.

In this connection it is important to say: no matter how deplorable, no matter how repulsive this whole matter might be, *individual* sexual offences cannot be stamped out with just a

Medical Rape

stroke of a pen, it takes more for that to happen. With another area it is different: the state itself must not in any case be involved in sexually perverted behaviour. *That* involvement could in fact be brought to an end with a pen stroke.... But, it isn't. By not reacting, by ignoring the calls for change, by ignoring calls to wake up, this state, the one that does nothing, has made itself responsible for aiding sexual abuse and harassment. And, this is indeed a very serious crime.

'Each and everybody gets what he deserves. The one who thinks he can disturb the work with cheeky comments and answers, he has to take the consequences himself. The one who tries to be smart, who tries to fake allergies or who fills the urine pot to the brim just to irritate us, he will soon regret his actions. Especially those who laugh at the start will shake when the call comes to pull down the pants. Then it will be examined longer down there, and when he is bent forward it can last five seconds, but also fifty.... It also depends on each person's behaviour whether he will be allowed to pull his foreskin back himself or whether the doctor will do it for him. Remember, also the *number* of witnesses can be decided by her.... So take care. Every guy decide himself if he wants to leave with a head like a mature tomato or not.'

Secretary Erika D.

The KWEA as Napoleon's Heritage

In the middle ages belligerent encounters were commonplace, almost a 'natural' part of life. Therefore the various rulers, with help of a variety of local systems, made it obligatory for their subjects to either train and fight themselves or, if they were rich and powerful enough, to have somebody else to do it for them. However, common for most countries at this time was that trained soldiers were only brought together when the realm actually was being threatened by attack - or, of course, if their ruler had got the idea to strike himself.

In the following centuries rulers got the fundamental idea that their respective countries needed permanent armies, and in some cases navies, in order to 'protect their people' (it was of course more about protecting themselves, but that is another matter). In other words: also in peace time there should be an army standing ready - 'just in case'. This was the first step towards general conscription, and, in this 'modernisation' drive France was in the driver's seat, leading the way.

Another import step towards the later introduction of obligatory war service for 'all' men came from the military theoretician Dubois Crancé. In 1789 he declared in the national parliament that in post revolutionary France every citizen should not just be that, an ordinary citizen, but also a soldier. However, the problem was that the conscription idea itself could not automatically be banded together with the idea of freedom and democracy, which, as we all know, had been the very basic theme of the revolution. No, many people were, to say the least, not enthusiastic about the idea. And, of course, it didn't make it better that also here, revolution or not, as everywhere else, some people would continue to be 'more equal than others'.

Of course, for those in power and with money there would be loopholes also within this new system. For example, if one had the financial means one could just hire a stand-in to march instead, and, of course, that was an opportunity used by many. That way the army continued to consist of people from the poorer parts of society - confirming the old truth that it is and continues to be the questionable privilege of the lower classes to kill and be killed in other (richer) people's wars.

Medical Rape

Of course, when building up a loyal, obedient army it is important to carefully consider every step that is to be taken. Here
we are back to what all this is about. The first step will be to
remove those who, for whatever reason, are to be seen as
less able to serve. For that purpose the *musterung* process
was established. Here the new recruit will be tested and evaluated - and, why not let him get a taste of his new future right
from the start? Yes, why not prepare him for what is to come?
Why not give him the first lesson on the road to unquestioned
obedience and total submission? Yes, why not?

How best to achieve quick subservience from new reluctant
recruits was quickly established. Why beat anybody up, leave
marks on his body and maybe harm the 'property' when other
methods could be even more effective? That was clear to
people already in those days. Already at this early time it was
clear to rulers how especially humiliated people quickly trans-
form into subservient subjects. The decision was, and it
seems like it came from Napoleon himself, every new recruit
had to present himself stripped naked for the *musterung*.

In France this method of humiliation was allowed to continue
all the way into the sixties and the rule of President DeGaulle,
the former hero general. DeGaulle was the man who understood the impact this would have on young people - probably
because he had experienced it himself. For him it wasn't
difficult to see the humiliating part of it all. All right, *musterung*
and conscription was to continue for many years, until it was
all finally abolished in 2001, but young people were at least
from then on allowed to keep their underpants on.

In Germany the word '*musterung*' was first heard in the
fifteenth century. It is probably derived from the Latin word
'monstrare' which means 'to show'. At this time the word
would then cover events where one's own potential armed
forces were counted and where it was decided how many
men one would have for the next 'crisis'. Not least, rulers were
here given an opportunity to see how well armed the soldiers
were.

This way soldiers were chosen for coming battles. It was
about finding the strongest, best and... holiest, but, and this is
important, there were no stripping and humiliation as part of
that. However, just like in France, this would change, and the

Prussians would take the lead. After all, they were experts in obedience and any method helping that to improve even further was welcome.

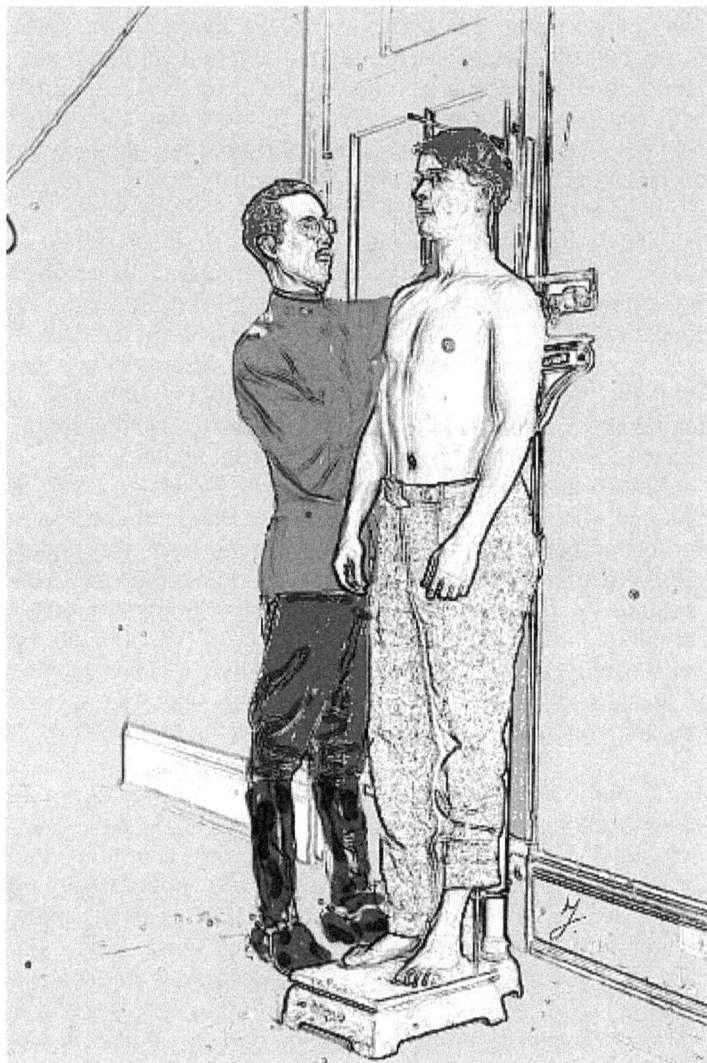

So it was that new soldiers started to have to present themselves naked before entering service for the mother land. If

Medical Rape

not before, at least during the German-French war 1870-71 this was the way things were being done. In the written instructions from those days it is clearly written: 'by the *musterung* the conscript while protecting his sense of shame has to present himself totally naked.' From that time and onwards this is now general practice. However, the instructions never explained how the conscript should 'protect his sense of shame' and what they actually meant with that. If they really were that concerned, why did they subject these young people to that degrading treatment?

Thereafter it became 'normal' that new recruits were paraded naked in front of doctors, officers and even civilians. However, there were short intervals of decency as well. The first was during the Weimar Republic (the post 'Great' War German republic) as the conscription, due to the Versailles accord from 1919, was abolished. But, that state of peace would of course change with the coming to power of Mr Hitler. With him and his Nazi cohorts the conscription and with that the *musterung* were re-introduced and continued in the same way as it had been conducted before - all leading to not only another horrible war but also to the second peaceful non-conscription period. Yes, again after World War II the people and its leaders - and more than anything else the winners of the war - had had enough of conscripted German forces and their belligerent exploiting leaders.

The risk somebody would be tempted to start a new war should now be curtailed, and as part of this precaution a new democratic constitution was introduced. This constitution was special because it was meant to be absolute, not to be tampered with and it was meant to secure the freedom of the people. It was meant to give to every (law-abiding) citizen in the country total freedom in life. On top of that a total de-militarisation of the country should follow to secure peace for the future. However, nothing lasts forever, and soon cries for a re-building of the armed forces were heard.

'A democracy needs an army in order to defend the freedom,' it was now stated, and, as a consequence of that, in 1956 the Constitution was changed with the introduction of the *'Wehrpflichtartikel'* (article of conscription). Mostly older men had now again, for the umpteen time in history, decided over future freedom, or rather future lack of such, for coming generations of male successors. This law should now affect all future male citizens in the Federal Republic of Germany.

In communist East Germany it was about the same - just much more oppressing, humiliating and... horrible.

'It wasn't easy to be naked in front of this man. It was indeed a weird feeling to stand there like that in front of a complete stranger. I had come for my second examination and this doctor again examined testicles and foreskin, as they had already done once before. He also wanted to have a quick look at my anus, and I allowed him to. At the end I was found "able".

'For me it was service as a conscientious objector in the civilian social sector. As I was to start there I had to attend one more examination - again more or less the same procedure. As before, nothing was left unattended; everything was done: heart, blood pressure, squatting and all the rest. After that, pants off and she went straight for my private parts....

'Sure, I do ask myself why it must be that important also for the civilian authorities to check my penis. Could be that you would get piles from too much sitting, but definitely not phimosis....'

Benedikt M.

Medical Rape

'I am Sure There is Some Humiliation Involved'

Today *musterung* of young men liable to the law of conscription is taking place in special draft centres, *Kreiswehrersatz-ämtern, KWEA*, and has changed into individual presentation. However, what is still there is the demand for the young person to present himself naked and what is even worse than in the past: it is no longer a ritual among men. Today the young men are mainly checked and controlled by all-women-teams.

> 'My third and last *musterung* experience was for me very embarrassing, as (once again) both anus and foreskin were controlled by a woman. This is for me nothing but sexual abuse, as these examinations are approved by the state, i.e. duty, and because one cannot get away from it. Of course, as an inexperienced young boy/man you haven't got the courage to refuse. You are made to believe that there is no option.'
>
> Serkan Ö.

This way the *musterung* practice under cover of a one-sided absurd interpretation of equal rights for woman has turned itself into the most obvious (though consistently denied) form of reversed sex discrimination. It has also turned itself into an attractive work place for those with certain interests.... After all, there will always be people who are more than happy to use such a chance to grab power over others and see them being humiliated and exposed.

'As I begun working as a medical secretary in a draft office, I wasn't familiar with what *"musterung"* actually was, at least not in details. The first three years I was there I worked for one specific male doctor and nothing exciting really happened. The closest to something thrilling could be situations like when a young man came into the room and didn't know what actually would happen. One could read the anxiety and insecurity in their eyes. When they saw me they probably thought: "oh, a woman!"

'But, the boys were always taken behind a screen for the more "special" examination, and the only thing I could hear was "please remove your pants"; "please cough;" and "do you have any problems?" Thereafter the doctor and the youngster came back out again. There was nothing there for me to see. The only excitement was what was in my fantasy.

'A year ago the male doctor was swapped with a female, forty-two years of age. This new doctor performs the examinations so that I can follow it all. First I found that embarrassing myself and avoided to watch. That has, however, changed. Today I do follow it all. If the guy is good-looking it is for sure quite arousing.... Very often it also seems like the doc and I have the same taste. Normally the examinations of the private part takes not much more than a minute or two. However, sometimes it can take two to five minutes. When that happens it is really about showing who is in charge.

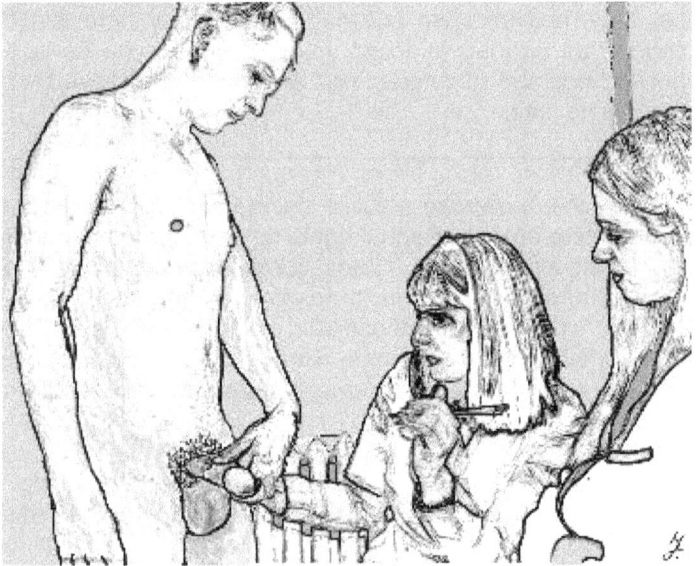

'All right, we do see a great number of both big and small penises, and we see lots of different testicles and backsides, but what arouses me most nowadays is the humiliation itself of the young man - to watch them when they have to pull down their underpants, bend forward and spread. Yes, the most exciting moment is when the doctor tells them in her firm voice: "turn around, spread your legs out and bend forward." Many just look totally bewildered. Sometimes they look over

Medical Rape

to me as if they ask themselves: "oh, and she is watching." When the penis get stiff as the doc examines the backside some also get red faces. When that happens, if not before, then I can actually feel a bit sorry for them. Yes, for sure, a bit humiliating it is. But, after all, these are the instructions; these are the rules.

'I can't help it, but I am quite fascinated by all this. I mean, at school and among their friends many of these youngsters will try to impress and play the big guy. But here, when stripped totally naked, they are just terrified docile little chaps.'

'Was it really necessary to put me through these humilia- ting, degrading examinations, and all in the presence of fe- male assistants and secretaries? That way they robbed me of the happiness in life which I, after lots of adversities, fi- nally had found just before these people got their hands on me.'

Niclas E.

Jeanette is one of those for whom it at least in the beginning was a little bit unpleasant to participate. 'I was assistant in San-Bereich,' she wrote in an internet forum. 'There the new recruits during their first week of service are examined just like by the *musterung*. They wait in track suits. For the me- dical they then have to strip down to the socks. That means, in that job one could see quite a few bare bums the whole day long. The doctor who was thirty-two at the time and privately quite a nice character surprised me with her insensitive style of examination. Yes, I did find it unpleasant when a grown up man, completely naked in front of two women, had to have his penis checked and foreskin pulled back. It was indeed quite crazy. She would stand there right in front of the guy, moving his penis to the right and to the left.... One could probably say she had another sense for privacy than most others - at least then it was about the privacy of others, or lack of such....

'First long time after I had left this place it became clear to me what a nightmare these examinations must have been for those exposed to it. At the time I didn't realise it; for us it was just seen as something natural and as a daily routine. Today, five years later, I can fully understand the anger shown by so many people.'

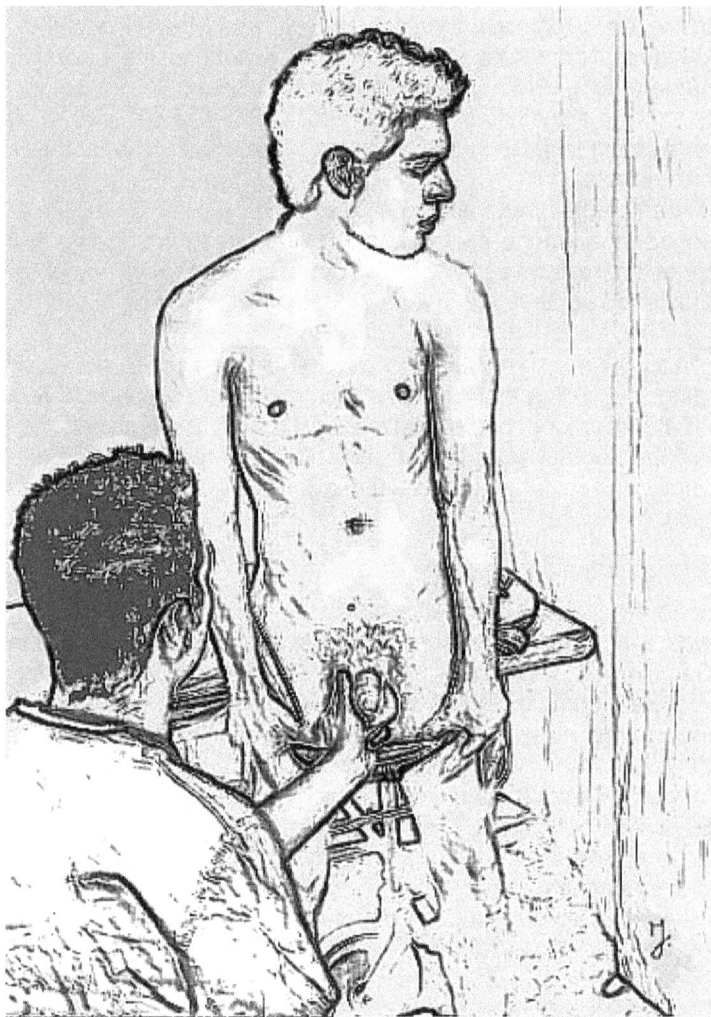

Of course, while some people in paid work can be allowed to humiliate others as they please (and enjoy that), the whole thing might cause lifelong suffering for the victims. Unfortunately, it seems like the state accepts that. In fact, it seems like nobody cares. A secretary puts it like this: 'what's the problem? After all, conscription is written into the constitution. I cannot imagine that it can be allowed just to be removed. I mean, if it was, then it would be unconstitutional. The *musterung* is part of that, and therefore it is right. After all, before I started to train for my job, I also had to go to the doctor. I couldn't just refuse that, and if I had I would have been without job. No, as I see it, there is a lot of whinging for nothing here.'

Has this woman forgotten that in a not too distant past there was no voting right for women? That was the law, so what was the problem? Why was it that that necessarily had to be changed? Only because the world has changed? Was it because *both* men and women in the modern world rightfully must have a right to freedom and dignity? Was it because men and women, at least in theory, must be equal before the law?

'It is unfortunate that the *musterung* doctors in their important and responsible examination work on a regular basis, as you must be aware of through some internet sites, are exposed to unfair accusations and insinuations. Therefore I am sure you will understand that when it comes to the necessary protection of the doctors against defaming accusations the use of screens must be seen as counter-productive. (...) It is not right to talk about exposure or humiliation.'

Minister of Defence Dr Franz Josef Jung

Lars G Petersson

A Very Special Interest

So what is this all about then? I think it must be something
deeper than just an inherited military perversion from the (Victorian) time of Emperor Wilhelm, a perversion which has been
seen in other countries as well. I think there is something
more behind it, and I think it is this: a perverted national interest in checking (other) people's genitals - under (real or felt)
duress, if needed or not.

> 'When it comes to the control of my genitals I fear most of
> all that I might get an erection. The thought of standing
> there stripped naked in front of a doctor and her assistant, I
> find extremely humiliating and embarrassing.'
>
> Sven F.

I have lived and worked in five different European countries,
including Germany. Most of the time I have worked in the
health service. When I compare my experiences I repeatedly
find myself back at the same issue: in Germany there seems
to be a very special interest in the genitals by most any medical examination or treatment; it seems like a reason for asking
people to strip can always be found. In the civilian area this
interest is probably focused on the female sex, at least when
it comes to adults.

It really makes me angry to know that there among medical
and caring staff are quite a few people who in these kind of
jobs have found a safe haven for perverted sexual fantasies
and sick longings for (sexual nature) power over other human
beings. Unfortunately, there isn't much focus on this huge
problem; I was about to claim that there is none, but that isn't
true either. Though it isn't much, there is indeed some, and it
comes from a very important place. All right, we have to go to
another (partly) German speaking country to find it, and it is
some time ago since the call first was heard, but yes, there it
is: under the decree 'no woman shall ever stand naked in
front of a doctor' the Medical Association in Basel has declared that the 'scope of sexual abuse in doctors' surgeries and
in hospitals is shocking.'

'Please, remove bra and knickers as well,' it is, according to
this medical association, repeatedly heard by the doctor, and

106

the same group of colleagues goes on to state that 'it is important to say that the removal of both of these garments is practically never needed'.

Because of this 'alarming situation' (as they have called it themselves) the association started a campaign to tidy up among their own black sheep and stop them from abusing their patients. No, a woman should never have to stand stark naked in front of her doctor, they declared, and, in order to achieve improved behaviour, a clearly written instruction was issued.

According to the association abuse is happening on a daily basis. An example of this is what happened to Claudia M. from Bern. 'We were alone in the consultation room as the doctor told me to get undressed. OK, I took of the sweater. However, then he also asked me to remove the bra.'

To put it mildly, that irritated Mrs M. After all, she had only come for a cold. Nevertheless, she did as she was asked and took her bra off as well, and after that the GP listened to her chest. Claudia M. felt bad about it all and did have the courage to ask if this really was necessary. 'It cannot be done in another way,' was the answer.

But no, it mustn't be like that. In GP surgeries and hospitals patients must be able to let themselves be examined without also having to have the feeling they are playing a part in a sexual play-doctor game. Doctors, whether male or female, who have such special interests should rather go somewhere else to have them satisfied. As we know well, it is absolutely possible to listen to a chest without having to remove the bra - just as it is possible to perform so many other examinations without having to strip the patient. All right, to help the abusive doctors control themselves, let us listen to their decent and devoted colleagues.

'It is clear that correct treatment starts before the patient finally meets the doctor. Often the staff wants the patients to wait undressed for that, and this must be refused. In the consultation room the patient is to be fully dressed when discussing the problem with the doctor. Ninety percent of a diagnosis can be made out of the history-taking alone. A patient shall never be fully undressed; there is no need for that. Only the area that is to be examined needs to be uncovered, nothing else.'

Lars G Petersson

In this context it is indeed remarkable also to read what Psychiatrist Werner Tschan, leader of a clinic for sexually abused patients (yes, such one exists), says: 'the "interested" doctor would specifically pick patients who are less able to defend themselves against voyeurism, people who are insecure and who would let themselves be manipulated. Therefore it is important to stop an examination if one feels the situation is turning unpleasant.'

Finally, as this problem seems to be much bigger than ever expected, the doctors at the medical association in Basel have worked out strict instructions for their colleagues. Therein, they clearly point out what kind of undressing is needed for specific medical examinations, and by doing so they go into remarkable details, which in itself shows the magnitude of the problem. They also address other ethical matters such as the patients' right to decide themselves what is to be done to them. 'For example, by a routine examination the doctor must always *ask* whether or not the patient also wants to have the genitals examined.'

This all sounds very good, but, yes there is a 'but' with all this: it is all solely about *women*. Of course, young men are not part of this concern for dignity and protection. They are just not mentioned. Obviously they can continue to be humiliated and exposed to degrading treatment, or so at least it seems. However, I have confidence that the doctors in Basel have just forgotten these people and that they are well intended and not gender biased. Still, it is indeed unfortunate.

It is unfortunate as the consequences of these young people being constantly forgotten can turn out to be extremely serious for hundreds of thousands of men's future health. For example: would you think the men in the following examples would ever volunteer to go to a doctor again, whoever he or she might be? Would you think they would ever dare run the risk of another assault?

Medical Rape

Jürgen's Experiences

'As a soldier one is supposed to defend the freedom of one's country and its citizens,' Jürgen said immediately after we had introduced ourselves. 'As a member of this society myself I think it is reasonable also to expect not to be excluded from the same freedom I am expected to fight for. However, I have realised that I am. Immediately after reaching adulthood, no matter if peace or war, as a male person one is no longer free: one can be taken over by the state and be used to practically whatever they want. Misused I would say - abused.

'I woke up this morning and felt pressure in my chest. I had had another night mare. It has been like that now for almost three years. I keep thinking about what happened. However, those who did it to me they will most likely never know about my suffering. And, even if they did, it is unlikely they would care.'

Pascal T.

'I would like to tell you about my experiences as they have remained with me in my head ever since. In 1999, as I was only seventeen, I was called up to attend *musterung*. I had heard quite a lot of nasty stories about it: one has to strip down to nothing, and the genitals will be thoroughly checked and controlled. I had also heard that the young person, standing completely naked, has to bend forward and have his anus inspected. In books from earlier times I had seen the same, so I thought, there must be at least something about it. But, to be honest, I couldn't really believe it was true. After all, people talk so much.

'No matter what, as I left for the draft office that morning, I was quite anxious about what would happen to me. Mr Petersson, as we both know why we are discussing this, I will save some time, leave all other details such as hearing, sight and all that aside and go directly to the point: I was called into an examination room by a female doctor. In there was another woman as well, a secretary. I looked around and saw a screen and felt a bit relieved.

'But, I wouldn't get away that easy. After the doctor had asked a few question about all and sundry, she pointed with her finger in the direction of the screen. I was told to go behind there, get (completely) undressed and come back out to the scales.... All right, now we were there. Now I should have to show myself stark naked in front of these two women, one of whom not much older than myself. I was terrified, and worst of all was that something started to happen between my legs....

'Yes, as I got undressed there behind the screen, I could feel a slight erection that I couldn't manage to suppress. I got extremely nervous. The two ladies would of course stare at my dick as soon as I came back out, and I didn't know what to do. I was about to panic.

'"Please, come back out," the doctor called. I must have had a face like a tomato as I quickly made my way to the scales. I could see how the secretary looked at me with a smile on her face. I cannot think about a more embarrassing situation to be placed in.

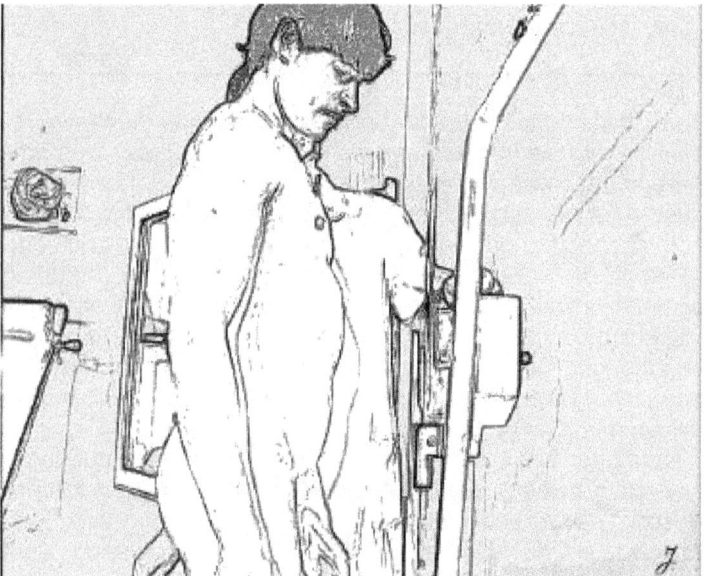

'Then I was weighed and had to stand with my back to the wall to have my height measured. All the time the secretary looked in my direction, while writing down the numbers dictated by the doctor. After that the doctor squatted in front of me with the words "now I will examine the genitals". Still this day I cannot get this picture out of my head. I find it extremely humiliating what they put me through. In fact, the part with the secretary was the worst of it all: I was so taken up by her watching that I hardly noticed the doctor. At least not till the moment when she asked me to turn around, bend forward and spread the buttocks with my hands....

'I couldn't believe it. It felt like all blood rush to my head. But, in that situation, what could I do? I had absolutely no courage to voice a protest, so I did what I was told.

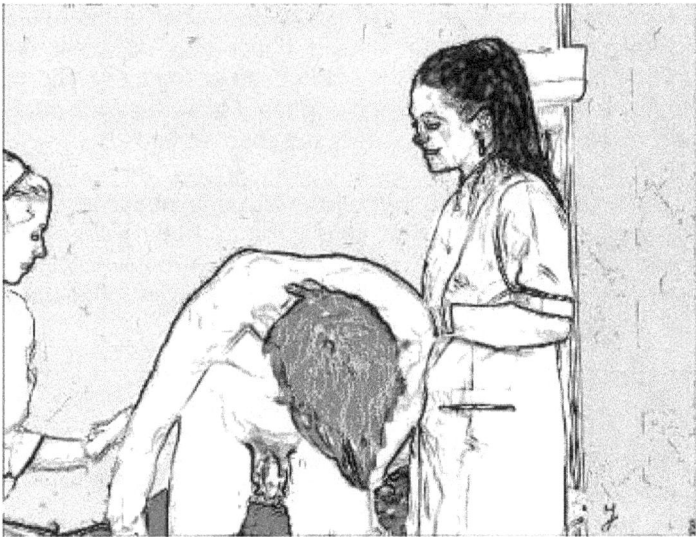

After a little while I heard the doctor say: "you can now get dressed, and please wait outside". Very quickly I got behind the screen, got my under pants on and rushed out of the room. What I had heard before I went for the *musterung* was true. I knew that now. When I think back on that day I feel so ashamed. All right, I had known fairly well what I had to expect. I cannot say I was surprised. But, that hadn't helped me. You cannot prepare yourself for such degradation.

'Many young people today are quite confident and outspoken. But I think, when they stand there in their Adam costumes in front of the ladies then they might be a bit less confident. As I was there for the *musterung* I remember a few wellbuildt young men in the waiting room. Also they would most likely have let them do what they wanted with them. Also these strong guys were most likely scared to bits. But, as things are, afterwards it will all be "forgotten". Afterall, nobody would like to be seen as a whinger; nobody would like to be rediculed and laughed at.

'Yes, that's how I look at it, Mr Petersson. And, of course, all this I have told you anonymously,' Jürgen said at the end of our conversation. 'Yes, we will never meet again, therefore, and only therefore, I have talked so openly about my deepest feelings. After all, one feels shame even if one has done nothing wrong. I really hope that other young men in the future will have the courage I didn't have. I hope they will speak out before it's too late. I hope they will refuse letting these people do the same to them as they did to me. I hope they will decline to become new victims. Life is too short for that.'

'To present oneself like that for the ladies is indeed embarrassing. However, worst of all is if the part being checked gets out of control and starts to grow.... What would be extremely embarrassing for one person can then of course be very amusing for the others.'

Guido Q.

Medical Rape

Peter Breaks his Silence

I met Peter a late afternoon in a *bierkeller* close to Hamburg Central Station. I had got to know him through the internet, and now he had agreed to meet for a chat.

Though this step out of anonymity had been extremely difficult for this man, though he had needed weeks to consider whether or not he would go along, now, at last, he had gathered enough mental courage to discuss his difficult memories with another person - so to say put it all into spoken words. A very long time these things had now plagued him. 'Why did my country do this to me?' that was the question he for years had kept asking himself.

'Thinking back, most of what I remember has something to do with what they did to my bollocks,' Peter began - hesitating, as he looked out of the window to the people rushing in and out of the station.

'"All right let us have a look," the doctor said after he had brought me behind a screen. It probably had taken no more than thirty seconds before we both came back out again. I was happy his secretary had seen nothing of that. Of course, the fear more than anything else was to get an erection. I felt relieved.

'Then I decided to do civilian service as an alternative to soldiering. The induction examination for that service took place in the so called *Gesundheitsamt*, a civilian state medical institution. There it was a bit different. My medical history was taken and blood tests were made as I was fully dressed (isn't that fantastic, authors comment). However, for the medical examination itself I had to completely strip. That was extremely embarrassing as it was in presence of not just a female doctor but also a female assistant. After that I was examined as at the musterung. She took her time, and, at one time, without warning, she just grabbed my penis and pulled back the foreskin. She was quite rough, and it was even painful. It was horrible to stand like that in front of these ladies.

Finally, after she had thoroughly checked my testicles, she asked me to turn my back to her and bend forward as deep as I could. That was for me just a mortifying experience, absolutely horrible. Nobody had ever done that to me before. I could really feel how the blood rushed up in my head; I must have been red as a tomato. After that I was allowed to get dressed.'

As I listened to Peter's story, it struck me how similar they all are. The day before another man had told me his story on the phone. Horst, that was his name, did not want to meet up personally. The shame over what had happened to him was too great. But on the phone he managed to tell his story.

'My *musterung* has stayed with me as an awful memory,' was his first hesitant words. But thereafter the ice was broken and he could hardly be stopped. It was very soon clear to me that this man had waited for years for somebody who would listen to him, somebody with whom he could feel safe, somebody who would take it seriously what he was about to tell, somebody who would not ridicule or laugh at him.

In this way one story sounds like another. By e-mail somebody with the name Herman wrote to me: 'we were ten guys in the room and were told to strip down to underpants and shoes. We were then called in separately to the examinations. In the examination room a woman sat behind a computer opposite the doctor who was a man. First it was all 'normal'. Then, however, as I thought it was all over, I was told to pull down the pants to the knees. The doctor pulled on gloves and got up from his chair. As he had finished to handle the scrotum, I was told to turn around and bend forwards. I did as he told me. After another short time I heard him telling me to turn back again. Having done that I noticed that he already sat on his chair and that I had been exposed in that position to the secretary.... As I after that was asked to pull back the foreskin I felt like running out.

'As my brother told me about this one day I was shocked. I didn't have a clue as to what they did in there. I thought they were just checking the physical ability for military service, if people were fit and able. But that? No, that's perverted. If my brother hadn't had so much trust in me as he has, then I think he never ever would have told anybody. Today I understand him better when it comes to certain matters.'

Martina N.

Medical Rape

For Boris it was about the same. Just like so many others he finds it horrible that also two female assistants had been present in the room. 'I still cannot understand what it was all about. Are they all perverts by the *Bundeswehr* (the armed forces)?' he asked me, as if he actually expected me to be able to answer that question.

'First I had to strip down to the underpants and do ten push ups and twenty squats. After that pulse and blood pressure were measured. Then my back was checked and thereafter 'it' came. For that I was asked to stand on a marked place on the floor with my back to the ladies. Why I had to stand right there I still ask myself. I continue to speculate about what could have been the reason. Could it really have been a hidden camera pointing at that spot?

'As the doctor now asked me to remove my underpants and lift up 'a leg' (as I understood it) I was totally gobsmacked.... After first having refused, I caved in (threats with 'consequences'...) and did what I was told. Now it became extremely embarrassing for me: I did not only stand there totally naked, I had also misunderstood his orders. The German word he had used can sort of be 'interpreted'.... So there I stood on one leg, and they all laughed. He had meant my penis. I will never forget what they did to me that day.

Achim's *Musterung*

'Twice I had to attend the draft examinations,' a young man, Achim, told me. This is his story: 'part of the *musterung* I already had behind me as we sat there in a kind of waiting room. On and off people passed us walking in and out of different rooms. Almost everybody who passed looked at us. We were almost naked, only dressed in underpants. It was quite a weird feeling; it felt like an eternity in there. As the others, one at a time, were called in to the doctor's room, I noticed it was a woman.

'Finally it was my turn. It was quite a big room and in a corner sat a secretary. I noticed she was very young and so was the doctor - probably in her early thirties. She was good-looking, and that made me fear I would get an erection. The atmosphere was unfriendly, and, of course, none of them introduced themselves. Without any introduction whatsoever the doctor just asked me to go behind the screen and get undressed. I did what I was told and totally ashamed and stark naked I stepped back out from the screen.

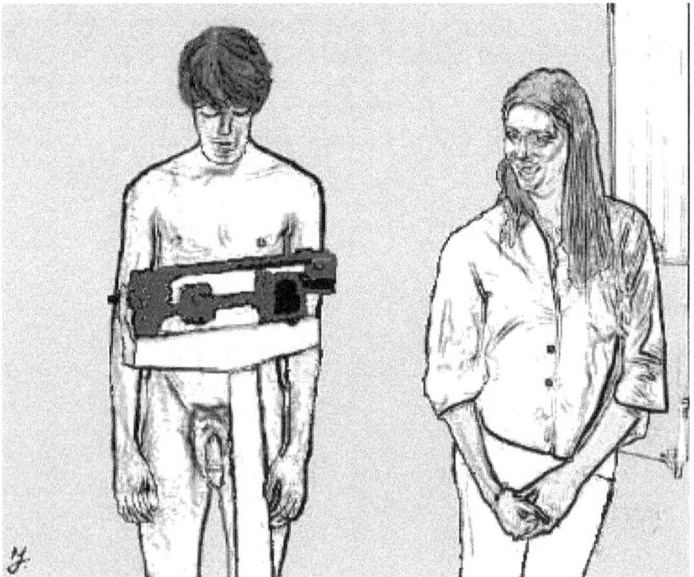

Medical Rape

'Before, in another room, I had already been weighed totally naked. Now I was to walk back and forth so that she obviously could have a look at my body stature. Some other examinations then followed, before she squatted in front of me and grabbed my testicles. Now I was asked to cough, and thereafter to pull back the foreskin. As I did so she was obviously not happy with the result and demanded it to be 'all the way back. please'. I must have had a totally red face as I could feel the heat in the cheeks, but, fortunately, I did not get a stiff. That must have been because of the shock - or maybe because all the blood had rushed up in the head....

'Thereafter I was asked to turn around, bend forward and spread my buttocks with my hands. I think she spent at least half a minute looking into my backside with a torch before she finally announced that everything was 'okay'.

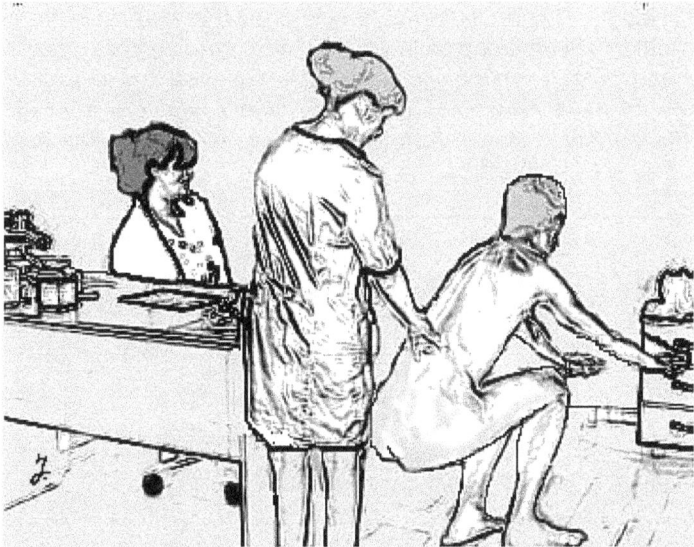

'After that it was time for the 'fitness test'. I first had to lay on a couch in the corner to have pulse and blood pressure measured. Then, still stark naked, I was 'asked' to do twenty squats before returning to the couch for another measuring. After that she waited about a minute. This time felt as an eternity. My blood pressure was 'quite high', I was then told, and she started to wait for it to fall. Shortly after she then repeated the measuring one more time and commented the result with: 'you are probably a bit nervous' (most likely the understatement of the year). After that ordeal I was allowed to get dressed and go to the next station.

'As I had expected, I was asked to come back next year. I will only say a few words about that experience: this time three women were present as I fully naked had to do squats and spread my buttock so that they could check my anus. It was extremely unpleasant. It is all just sickening.'

'The whole thing makes me so bloody angry. So many horrible thoughts keep popping up, no matter how much I try keeping them at bay. Why is it that I had to be part of that? After all, I am a human being, and also I have constitutional rights - at least I think so....

'Had I just been aware of how to protect myself, then they wouldn't have been able to play with me like that. Had I been what I am now I would have opened my mouth; I would have refused. That would have saved me from all this suffering. Now I have to try and live with my memories. They are impossible to change.'

Klaus R.

Medical Rape

Ibrahim's *Musterung*

This far we have probably seen a traditional ethnic German youngster as victim of this abusive behaviour. However, Germany has a large immigrant population, many of those with Turkish background. So what about them? What about those young people with a Muslim background? Nowadays many of these will be having German passports and citizenships meaning they too will be subjects to the conscription law - and to the *musterung*, inductions and discharge medicals.

If it is difficult for ethnical German young men to speak about their experiences with the strip examinations, how will it be for those with other backgrounds? With whom can they talk? Traditionally, when it comes to Turkish Muslim families, all subjects which could have anything to do with sex are considered taboo - and, no question, forced striptease and grabbing out after other people's genitals would come under that. Therefore, the chance that young people from these groups would be actively supported by the older generation must be considered as being fairly slim. No, also here an exchange of experiences is only possible, if ever, with people who themselves have had the same experiences. However, one advantage the Turkish young man would have toward the ethnic German: he will not risk being a laughing stock. He will not be ridiculed. He will be understood.

But, there is another side to the coin as well: exactly this feeling of shame that might draw people together makes the whole issue into a complete taboo. Therefore this subject cannot be talked about in the community. This way this abuse also in these immigrant groups have developed into 'their common secret' - the secret they share with their tormentors. As I found it extremely important that this book also should contain opinions from these groups of 'new Germans', I decided to try and find someone who would be willing to share his experiences and thoughts with me. That was, to be completely honest, not an easy task. Finally, however, through friends of friends, I managed to find him.

Let us call this young man Ibrahim. We had agreed to meet in a coffee shop close to the central station in Düsseldorf, and there he was as I arrived, a likable twenty-five years old man with a friendly smile on his lips. As we, after a short initial conversation around Ibrahim's education and plans for the future, got on to the subject, he told me a story which in most details sounded like all others only slightly different. 'The examination was done by a male doctor; the female secretary to start with sat behind a desk.

'At this time I was only dressed in my underpants. I was asked all the usual questions about earlier diseases and/or medical problems. Thereafter I had to do squats and blood pressure and pulse were measured.

At the end I was then asked to remove the underpants. As I did so, the secretary got up from her chair with her notebook and parked herself right beside me.... As the doctor went on checking my genitals, she was staring directly at my private parts. I felt extremely embarrassed by this treatment and was relieved when it was all over.

Despite his experiences with this very special part of Germany Ibrahim identifies himself with the society in which he lives. 'For me the army was a good thing. I was away from my family and learned to manage on my own. That way I went through a personal development. If the time by the forces works like that then I would recommend it to others. But, they have to be able to go there with pride and come back out with pride.'

This far immigrant organisations are all remaining quiet about this issue, probably because they are not aware of the situation. Of course, their young people are just as quiet about what they have been exposed to as all others. But, will it stay like that? Precisely Muslim citizens, not least those of Turkish origin, are often blamed for not living up to the constitution's call for human rights and respect for the rights of the woman. Here one day there might be some very difficult questions for the authorities to answer....

Medical Rape

'Even on the Scales Underpants are Allowed'

An assistant calling herself Britt is telling this story from her work place: 'The examination of the private parts normally do not last longer than a few minutes. In order to protect the young people the doctors allow them to keep their underpants on until the last moment. Only at the end they have to strip totally naked.

'Normally the young people are able to pull back their fore-skin themselves. Therefore there is no reason to fear that anybody without warning will just grab the genitals; it's all done in a very sensitive manner. After the foreskin has been tested for its function, the rest of the penis is thoroughly exa-mined for defects which can cause problems by urinating and intercourse. At this point the doctor also looks out for signs of sexually transmitted diseases. After that she checks the tes-ticles for cancer, examines the groins for hernia and the anus for piles and that's it, it's all over.

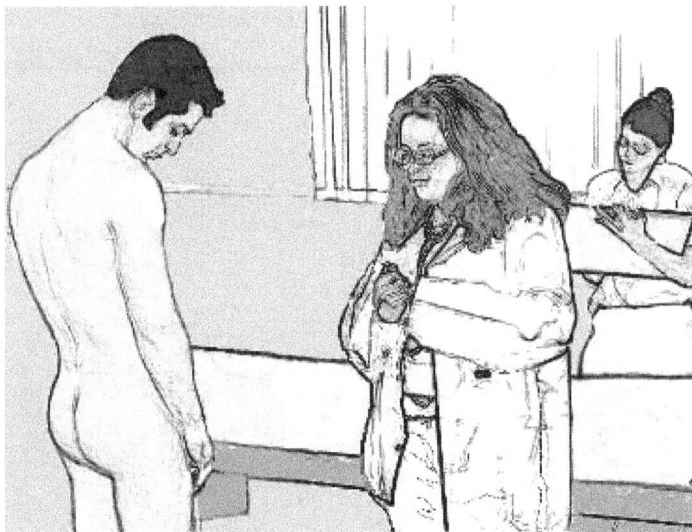

'The dignity by this process is protected at all time, as the youngsters are called in one by one and no conscript is allo-wed to see what is being done with another. The genitals and backsides are only seen by the doctor and her assistants. Nobody else will be there. In fact, even when they are being weighed, they are allowed to keep their underpants on.

'It is true, nakedness is limited to the most necessary; we respect thoroughly that people can be embarrassed. It is also so that those who perform the examinations have long experience in their jobs; they have been psychologically trained, and, not least, they have seen hundreds and again hundreds of totally stripped men before. It's nothing new to them. The youngsters who have to endure these examinations can rest assured about that. So there is no need to be ashamed.

'I can only give this advice to the one who under no condition wants to spend the entire examination totally naked. Put on normal underpants or at least boxer shorts and bring with you precisely what is said in the letter. I made the error to put on so called skater shorts. As the doctor then said that I should remove everything except the underpants, I couldn't as I had none on.... The result was that I was just told to remove it all. This way she conducted the entire examination, everything, with me completely naked.'

Lutger B.

Medical Rape

Letter to the Minister

Dear Minister Jung (and subsequently Minister Guttenberg),

I write to you as part of research for my new book. The subject of this work will be the violation of young men's right to dignity in the Federal Republic of Germany with particular stress on the forced military examinations of genitals and anuses, which most young people consider extremely humiliating.

For some months by now I have been collecting background information and have conducted interviews with affected people. Unfortunately, by doing so I have realised that the problem seem to be much worse and much more serious than I had ever anticipated. The numerous stories of serious abuse which have come to my knowledge have convinced me even more about the importance of this project. I have come to realise that something urgently must be undertaken to protect young people in your country against further ill-treatment. This is extremely important as many of the people I have talked to in the process of researching this book have suffered for years as a result of what they have been exposed to during military medicals.

Horrors around humiliating military medicals are nothing new. Horrible stories have been told from the eras of the Emperor (i.e. Victorian time) and the Nazis, but, in fact, they have never stopped coming in. Yes, during all the modern military history nakedness and humiliation have been walking hand in hand with the military establishment in the process of training new recruits. There must be a reason for that, and for sure there is. Forced nakedness is a very effective weapon in the process of creating submissive, obedient soldiers. It is the first simple but very effective step in a long line established to break down resistance. This way young men are changed into subservient, obedient soldiers, soldiers who do what they are told - including rape.

We cannot change the past, but, and this is important, we *can* try and prevent horror from repeating itself in the future. There are very good reasons for that. First, the world has changed. As minister of defence I am sure you do not want that kind of soldiers in your troops any longer. They don't belong in modern defence forces. Second, young people in your country, no matter if conscripted or enlisted, must have the same constitutional rights to be treated with respect and dignity as all other people in society. Today, all these years after the end of the Nazi rule and the disappearance of the Communist East German dictatorship, nobody should be allowed to be humiliated by the state.

Of course, this should be obvious, but still, in your country it seems not to be. This is indeed remarkable. After all, when it comes to these abusive military-related medicals the victims are to be counted in millions.... In fact, we talk about the ongoing abuse of half of the growing-up population. So how can it be allowed to go on like that? Probably this is the answer: embarrassment stops people from speaking out. And, young people quite frankly do not have the courage to defend themselves against this blatant abuse. Of course, it doesn't make it easier for them that their obvious lack of knowledge regarding their basic human rights often is shamefully used against them in order to mislead them into accepting things which other people never would go along with. Many young people thereafter spend years trying to (re)establish confidence and trust in the medical profession.

Not only is this medical abuse of young people allowed to be continued as usual, it has in the last decades got much worse. Nowadays, as a rule, completely naked young men are examined and evaluated for war service by *women* - and this in front of at least one more of the opposite gender, a secretary. This situation is by most young people seen as extremely humiliating and discriminating - not least because these people themselves are not liable for the same duties and because women who volunteer for the army are treated in a completely different and respectful way.

It might be that such a treatment as these young men are exposed to would have been a 'valuable' preparation for somebody joining a military dictatorship's armed forces, and it was most likely an excellent exercise before becoming a fully trained SS officer or *Wehrmacht* soldier. But, I am not that sure about its relevance when the individual is to serve a peaceful twenty-first century European country. After all, we must today realise that we live in another time; we live in a united Europe, a modern age. We do not need violent rapists and torturers any longer (as if *we* ever did). In fact, they are not wanted. They are not wanted in the civilian society, and, important, they are not wanted by the military either.

No matter how one looks at this matter, it is nothing but a disgraceful scandal. Systematically to humiliate young people is a shame for the government of the Federal Republic of Germany and it is a shame for the entire German people. We are dealing with a very serious problem: how many young people have this far already killed themselves because the memories of the embarrassing treatment were too big a burden for them to bear? We don't know. However, one thing we do know is this: the social group in society with the by far highest rate of suicides is young males. In how many of all these cases have the German armed forces had a part to play? In how many of these cases have the 'play doctor games' played a part? We don't know, but it might be worth thinking about, especially if one is the minister ultimately responsible....

Testicular cancer can be fatal. Therefore it is important that young people are encouraged to check themselves *regularly* in order to detect any sign that could indicate problems. They should be taught how to do so by somebody competent - that is if they want to. That would be good for young men and their health, as this disease can occur at any time. Yes, as we all know, it is not so that a one-off forced examination at age 17-21 would solve the problem for ever. Much more likely is that nothing will be found. But, what about a month or a year later? If cancer *now* grows and remains undetected due to bad experiences from the *musterung* examinations, who will then be ultimately responsible? Who will be responsible for this person to miss out on life saving treatment?

It is indeed possible that young men would not even examine themselves because of the risk of detecting anything that could lead to a visit at the doctor's surgery. This way the forced examinations are not only to be seen as abuse of the privacy of young people, they can also lead to non-detection of serious disease. In the worst scenario they can lead to premature death.

- Is the state aware of its responsibility for this? Are you aware of your personal responsibility?

One could easily imagine the following situation: by a young man, who is being examined completely naked in the presence of two or three women, a lump is found in one of his testicles. Cancer? While standing there like that, he will then be told about this terrifying possibility. I find it absolutely shocking that this combination of total humiliation and being told of possible cancer can be allowed to happen....

- How can you allow this to take place? How would a young person ever come to terms with such an experience?

I am very interested in hearing your opinion also to the following questions:

Medical Rape

- What has young men's foreskin to do with the defence of Germany? I cannot understand why the Defence Forces are showing such an interest in the free movement of foreskins. Any reason? Please advise.

- Please explain, if the Ministry of Defence out of sheer kindness and concern wants to offer help in this area, why do its doctors not first ask the individual person whether or not he is interested in the offer?

- Could you please advise how these abusive examinations can be in line with Article 1 of the German Constitution (in which the state is obliged to protect its citizen's dignity at all time)? Note, there are no exceptions to this constitutional right of protection. Please explain the discrepancy between that fundamental law and the general practice within your department.

- Why do young men have to strip completely during the military examinations and why do these checks of their private parts have to take place in front of female assistants? Please explain.

- Why are these examinations very often repeated not just once but several times, also when the reason for a renewed *musterung* examination has nothing to do with the private parts? Seems like harassment to me.

- Why is the whole process repeated at the start of the service - including testicles, foreskin and anus - not only by the *Bundeswehr* but also by the civilian authorities? Can this be seen as anything but abuse?

Please, be aware of the following: haemorrhoids in young males are rare. Also, somebody who suffers from them would be very likely to look for a doctor of his own choice, one he would feel comfortable with. I can hardly believe that the very rare cases of piles by eighteen-year-old men in any way can defend forced examinations of the anus not only at the military *musterung* but also at the beginning and end of the service and sometimes also in between.

If the Defence Forces really are that concerned about young people's anal health, why do they not just ask the individual whether or not he has a problem, and, if so, if he wants help with it? And, why are they not 'concerned' about women's health in the same area? Precisely, why do they not also examine female *volunteer* applicants and staff for the same? After all, haemorrhoids by females are statistically much more frequent. A remarkable neglect of *their* health..... isn't it? Or should we just accept that the reason for these checks is something totally different? This is indeed a very important issue. Therefore, please answer following questions:

- On what medical evidence does the state base these forced controls of young men's back sides? 'Bend forward, spread the buttocks, have a look'.... In what medical literature can I find the evidence for the correctness of such an examination method? What are your people actually looking for? Allow me to say: this is indeed a very 'unusual' method of medical examination, one never seen in any medical text book.

Today all interventions that a clinician undertakes - examinations and/or treatments - must be evidence-based. Consequently, a clinician must be able to demonstrate that he/she bases his/her actions on current scientific evidence.

- Is there any medical evidence saying that soldiers with piles can put the defence of Germany in danger?

Medical Rape

- What is the real reason behind inspections of this part of the body? I can only see abuse. Do you have another opinion about this question?

I am confident that I am right when stating that the German defence forces have widely distanced themselves from methods used during the time of the Emperor and the Nazis. And, I am sure the armed forces today are not training their soldiers to become rapists. I am equally convinced that the ambition is to have morally secure and responsible soldiers to serve the country, people who are trained for modern times and modern needs. But, on that background it is for me impossible to understand that humiliating 'training' methods which originate in a dictatorial past are still allowed.

No question, hardly anybody who finds himself standing there stark naked in front of people whose orders he has to follow will have the confidence and strength to refuse to do what he is then told. If one is only seventeen it would be so much more obvious how difficult such a situation would be. But, to refuse having one's private parts exposed and examined like this should not even be necessary. After all, 'play doctor games' belong to childhood or to consenting adults. Under no circumstances should it be allowed to be a part of state-employed medical staff's daily work. Nobody should have to take part in 'play doctor games' by the doctor....

Many people - my research has clearly demonstrated - cannot come to terms with the memories of the military (and conscientious-objector related) examinations and the extreme humiliation which was part of it all. They continue to suffer mentally. Remember, at the time all this happens to a young man he is right in the middle of a very sensitive time of his development, also sexually.

Let me also remind you: as the minister ultimately responsible for what the armed forces and their medical services undertake in the name of the German nation you are under duty to act in order to protect the young generation as according to Article 1 of the Constitution. As Germany is a signatory of the European Convention on Human Rights, which *prohibits* degrading treatment (Article 3), you, as responsible minister, is also under obligation to see that your state employees comply with the most fundamental principles of decent human behaviour. If failing to do so you will be taking upon yourself a very big responsibility. Remember sexual abuse of defenceless, vulnerable young people is a criminal offence.

I am looking forward to your answer.

Yours Sincerely

Lars G Petersson

Originally this letter was written in German in January 2009 to Minister Jung. It was also sent to all MPs and all relevant bodies within the German political administration. After change of guards it was re-sent to the new minister of defence, Guttenberg, first in the original version and then, July 2010, also in an English version. This far I have not had a reply to questions asked.

Medical Rape

The Problem With the Oath

It is possible that practising medicine for some people has more in common with playing sex games and dominating defenceless people than treating diseases and alleviating suffering. But, it is difficult to see how these doctors then can link such activities with the oaths they once swore. Most likely they can't. In fact, the oaths seem to be forgotten; they seem to have lost meaning. Yes, it very often looks like some of these professionals never have sworn to 'give their life in service of humanity', or promised 'with all my ability (to) defend the honour of the profession.' Neither they can have sworn 'never to use the medical art contrary to the basic principles of humanity' nor 'to practise the profession with consciousness and dignity'. How can it otherwise be possible to behave oneself as if these oaths never have existed?

Indeed, there are here two very serious questions which need to be asked. First: can it really be allowed just to repeat these words as a parrot and thereafter just forget all about them? Second: if someone really *has* forgotten that he or she once has promised to 'show every human life respect', and, even if under threat, 'not to use the medical art in a way contrary to the principles of humanity', should this person then not just have to quit and leave the profession?

For sure, two completely different worlds are clashing. So what should doctors do when they find themselves in such a conflict of interests? The answer must be obvious: for anybody having promised to use their life in the interest of humanity there can be no doubt. There are no alternatives. There is only one way to go and that is out - leave. If anybody wants to be taken seriously and if he/she wants to remain faithful to the ethical standards of medicine then there are no alternatives, no other options. If one wants to work as a doctor one *has* to follow the oath of the own profession and not the one guiding an institution with a fundamentally different ethos.

From all this we can see that there cannot be any room for doubt regarding the duties of medical staff. First and foremost: the loyalty to the patient must always be the top priority - loyalty to the state must be second to that. Furthermore, a doctor has to follow the rules and regulations for his/her own profession and must stay independent of external pressure. That means, they are not allowed to undertake any duties which are not in line with the basic medical responsibilities they have to their patients.

> 'Before it was my own turn I had noticed that the last two boys leaving the examination room had done so with red faces. Already as we arrived in the morning they had appeared shy and anxious. Are they now suffering just as me, all these years after? Probably they are.'
>
> Jochen K.

As we have seen, there have been a number of national and international initiatives in order to regulate this area and secure patients' rights. German doctors have done their bit as well, and, as a result of that, a medical code of conduct (die *Berufsordnung*) has been adapted by the Medical Board in order to regulate its members' (i.e. all registered doctors') behaviour towards not only patients but also colleagues, other professional partners within the health service and, not least, the general public.

This *Berufsordnung* is there to defend the freedom and the reputation of the medical profession, and it is there to encourage good professional behaviour and discourage bad. And, that's good, isn't it? It definitely is. Not least it is good because with those regulations as support we do not need to *ask* for improvements, we can *demand* them. Yes, all that is good news for us and bad for the abusive doctors. And they, the latter, they are in for more: their situation is not exactly made easier by the military establishment itself. Believe it or not, even from that side, in their own code of conduct, we can call for support in our struggle for decency and dignity. More about that in the following.

All right, let us have a closer look at this and let us first read what the medical code's second paragraph says. Here we learn that 'doctors are conscientiously to perform their duties strictly in line with good medical ethic and humanity' and that 'they are not allowed to adopt or acknowledge any principle or consider any instruction which is not reconcilable with their duties or which in itself is irresponsible.'

Medical Rape

Yes, so it is, and already here doctors who work for the draft boards and for the civilian health offices dealing with the conscientious objectors will be in for trouble. But, those troubles will still come in second to those in store for the medical people who are working *within* the armed forces. In fact, they are making themselves guilty of even more breeches of rules and regulations, this time against the armed forces' own code of conduct.... If one soldier humiliate another - as he/she will do with perverted play doctor games - this will constitute such an offence. In this case the doctor and the helper cannot hide behind the usual excuses such as 'I just obeyed order' and 'I just did what I was told'.

No, it seems like the doctors within the forces do have serious problems to deal with. By accepting to do the jobs they are doing, they must not only have 'forgotten' or put aside their own medical code of conduct, but, on top of that, the German soldier's law as well.... That was indeed unwise of them, to say the least. As employees by the armed forces it is in fact their blatant duty strictly to follow this law. No, there is no excuse whatsoever for a medical doctor and his/her assistant (both technically soldiers) not to know that paragraph 11 in this law very clearly says that it is not a case of disobedience if an order which either has nothing to do with the service or would violate the human dignity is not obeyed. In the same way, but with even more force it is stated that 'an order is *not allowed* to be obeyed when a criminal offence (in this case a sexual assault in form of deliberate humiliation of a forced naked, dependent person who cannot defend himself) would be the outcome'.

Just as serious it would be not to know (and to honour) that, according to paragraph 12, the unity of the armed forces is 'due mainly to comradeship' and, particularly in this case, that it is a 'duty for all soldiers to honour the dignity, honour and rights of all comrades' (i.e. all other German soldiers). When a medical doctor then violates the dignity of her fellow soldier comrades by ordering them to turn round and spread their buttocks, it can be nothing but a very serious offence according to this paragraph - a clear step far over the boundaries of acceptable behaviour.

Furthermore, in paragraph 17 it is clearly stated that the behaviour of every soldier (in this case the doctors and their assistants) must not do damage to the reputation of the armed forces. Here one must be allowed to state that pornographic play-doctor-by-the-doctor games at least do not do much to *improve* the reputation of the institution.

No, one need not be a lawyer in a military court to understand that mass humiliation of one's own soldier 'comrades' is a serious offence against the soldiers' own law. Every single soldier *must* know that. Therefore I think it is all right to ask the question: have these people ever read all these texts? In fact, they should have. After all, they are under legal obligation to follow the rules, so I think it would be a very good idea if they started to make themselves familiar with the contents.

'First I had to strip down to my underpants (for hearing and eye tests...), then behind a screen to remove the last cover and back out to have the foreskin pulled back and forth and the testicles controlled. I was first deemed not suitable for war duty and sent home.

'Then, one year later, back again and once more a total striptease. This time they were two lady doctors to do the job. I stood there right in the middle of the room. Of course, the foreskin could have got stuck in the year that had passed, and the testicles might have disappeared, so again it was all checked carefully. After that I was 'asked' to turn around and spread the buttocks - all in front of their young female secretary.

'This second time the blood tests weren't quite right, or so they said, so on to some consultant and then back for one more show of all the same. It's all a circus, and the men are the clowns.'

Cornelius C.

Medical Rape

The Role of the Medical Boards

The armed forces, the *Bundeswehr*, have acknowledged that also their doctors as well as those working for the draft offices are legally obliged to comply with the medical code of conduct.

And, as far as I can see, no medical board - neither the federal nor the ones responsible for every individual state - has ever questioned this obligation either. Of course, it would have been difficult to explain if they had, but they haven't. Having realised that, we are then left with the question: why do these medical boards not get actively involved when breeches of the code are as obvious as they are. After all, it cannot have been the very first time they heard about it as in 2009 all states' medical boards formally, in writing, were asked by associates to me as well as by me to declare where they stand on this issue. They were asked not only to act in support of the young men (i.e. the 'patients') and protect them from medical malpractice, all of that definitely within the remit and responsibility of medical boards (see the example from Basel), but also, and here there can be no question regarding their duties, to protect those of their own members who while working in these institutions want to avoid breeching the oaths they once swore.

But, for whatever reason, none of these boards has shown the slightest interest in the issue. The most common way out of the dilemma has simply been to refer to their own 'limited responsibility' that prevents them from acting or making a statement. Indeed a fairly remarkable explanation.... an explanation that more than anything else looks like wishful thinking, one expressed by somebody who desperately wants to find a way not to be involved.

Precisely so, how can their responsibility in this area be limited? After all, *all* doctors are requested to be members of these medical boards. They all pay membership fees to them and cannot act in their profession if they don't. So how can the boards claim they cannot get involved when these members are required to perform unethical tasks by their employers? How can they claim it to be beyond their area of responsibility to protect their own members, those who want to work ethically? And, how can it be outside of their area of responsibility to defend parts of the general public against their own misbehaving members, those who *do not* want to work ethically? Indeed some interesting questions. Yes, why do they not want to get involved?

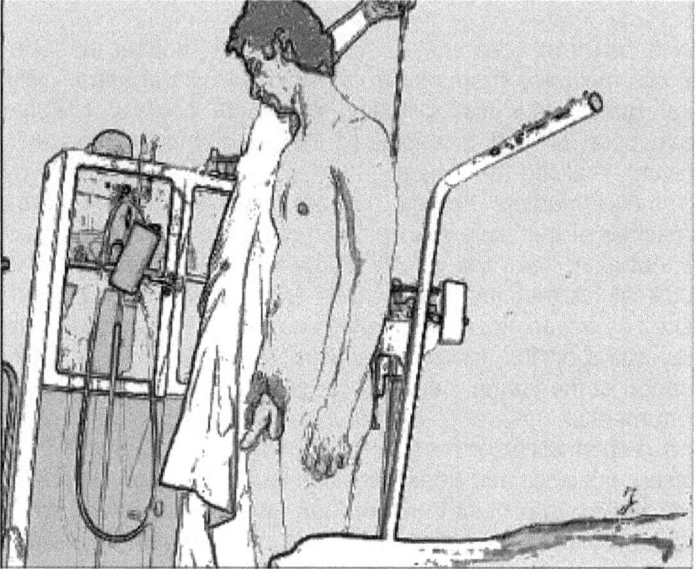

No matter what, the boards go far to get around this issue. They shun no methods. What is nothing but an *ethical* and *medical* matter they happily either refer to the Ministry of *Defence* or to the *military* ombudsman, or, alternatively, explain away themselves with 'smart' literal constructions like the one here: 'doctors who in compliance with their contracts are carrying out necessary examinations are not in breech with their professional duties...'. Yes indeed, rather inventive. Sounds good, doesn't it? But what about the *un*-necessary ones...? After all, that was what the question was about, wasn't it? No, not a word about that. Those 'examinations' were happily 'forgotten' - easiest so.

  The boards had other ways as well to get out of the pickle. They had other methods which, if necessary, could be used. An example of that could be like this: why not just claim that you 'understand' the question in another way than it was asked and then just construct your own answer that fits your own version of the original question. That's indeed clever, but, of course, it requires some effort and time, so in quite a few cases easier ways out were used: either the real question was simply ignored and some nonsensical lines were written which had nothing to do with the problem, or, as happened in most of the cases, they just didn't answer at all; they simply ignored the whole letter.

Interesting is that not only the smaller state boards but also the federal medical board, *'Die Bundesärztekammer'*, consistently has avoided to comment on this issue. As with their junior bodies in the states also this board has eagerly declared that the issue is outside of their responsibility.... Obviously, as must be my conclusion, if German doctors want to abuse their patients, the federal medical board won't get involved.... Indeed interesting, and shocking.

'The medical *musterung* examination generally takes place only in the presence of *one* third person (forensic principle). This system, which is also practised by civilian medicals, is independent of the gender of the examiner and/or the person being examined.'

Minister of Defence Dr. Franz Josef Jung, 2009

Lars G Petersson

The 'Forensic Principle'

So what is in reality this so called 'forensic principle' which seems to be so important for the Ministry of Defence and which so frequently is used in order to defend the abuse? To be honest, what is behind this so called principle, and where is it legally to be found? What is the background for it? What is it actually there for?

These are important questions to be asked as the former Minister of Defence Jung (on behalf of the ministry) in some of the responses to the criticism compares the whole issue to 'identical practises also in the civilian area'. This way he and his staff try to legitimise the forced exhibition of young naked men in front of female examination teams. This is of course an unbelievable abuse of a safeguarding system which in the civilian medical area (in England we would use the term 'chaperone') has been established to *protect* not only doctors but also patients. It was definitely not meant to make it *worse* to be a patient. It wasn't meant to add to the exposure and the vulnerability.

These are some facts: just as is the case with the British system of offering a patient a 'chaperone' when being examined by a doctor, the German version, the so called 'forensic principle', is not a law but (much better) just common sense. It is a well-intended initiative put in place to protect both patients and doctors: it protects the patient from abusive behaviour and it protects the doctor from false and unfair accusations. Used in that way it is indeed a very good thing. But, in fact, all this has very little to do with the term 'forensic'. The only likely explanation for the use of that word in this connection might be that the arrangement hopefully can prevent that the doctor's and his patient's first meeting in the surgery will be followed by a second in court - this time with 'chaperones' on *both* sides and a judge in the middle.

There are a few other things which also are seen as parts of this principle. First: before the examination the patient must be explained about all matters involved and all options. After all, it is her/ his body. Second: he/she is not to be undressed more and for longer time than is absolutely necessary for the procedure that is to be undertaken. And third: the assistant must be of the same gender as the person being examined.

Medical Rape

As we can see, most everywhere this principle of decency is recognised, everywhere except by the armed forces and their associated clinics.

> 'It can never be justified to talk about "exhibition" or "humiliation" when talking about the intimate part of the *musterung* examination.'
> Minister of Defence Dr. Franz Josef Jung 2009

November 6th 2009 there was a meeting for leading *musterung* doctors at the *Bundeswehr* medical academy in Munich. Among other issues the strip examinations and the genital and rectal checks on men in presence of all-female examination teams were discussed. What I know happened at this meeting I find shocking.

According to my internal sources leading Medical Director Bernhard Rymus from the defence administration, the *'Wehrverwaltung'*, verbally instructed his people that the screens during examinations of genitals and rectal areas must be removed altogether.

In some of the institutions and by some doctors (as far as I can see mainly by the few males) these *had* been used to protect the victims from being watched by female secretaries during the embarrassing parts of the examination. However, now the screens, according to Director Rymus, should be removed altogether, this way allowing the female assistants full access to follow in detail all stages of the examinations. The obvious and unhidden objective for this: any complaint would this way easily be rendered completely harmless. The witness' testimony would assure that. That the witness herself, solely by her presence, would constitute a very large part of the problem was not mentioned with a word. And, in no way it was discussed how to prevent the whole procedure from being what it is, a criminal abuse of power over defenceless young people. No, it wasn't about that; it was exclusively about how to prevent any complaint from being successful, and Rymus' instruction was of course meant to do the job.

To understand that Mr Rymus and his friends are dead serious about this last blow to young people's dignity we only need to have a look at this letter from Minister Jung:

'Unfortunately, as you will be aware of through some internet sites, the highly responsible *musterung* doctors again
and again are confronted with unfair accusations and
associations. I am sure that you will therefore understand
that the use of screens are counterproductive to the
necessity of protecting these doctors from undeserved and
defaming accusations.'

Minister of Defence Dr. Franz Josef Jung, 2009

Medical Rape

Abuse - 'Burglary into my Soul'

'For years I had managed to keep my experiences at the draft office fairly well "forgotten", Heinz S. declared to me as we sat there in a coffee shop, discussing a topic that was very much concentrated on his - this ten minutes before for me totally unknown man's - foreskin.

'However, then I came under suspicion by the police and my home was searched. I was devastated. I had no idea I had done anything wrong, and I hadn't. That I was totally innocent was also very soon obvious for the officers, who with a polite "sorry" left my flat. Yes, it had been a mistake, but now, after they had searched all my most personal belongings, I wasn't, as one would have expected, relieved: I was back at the draft office.... Again I felt I had been forced to show the authorities my most intimate parts. It had 'only' been my personal belongings this time, but it had felt like back there: 'remove all your clothes, strip.'

'After this day I was back with the lady doctors, and from now on I cannot free myself from the memories any longer. Now, in my mind, these people continue to visit me, and this makes it impossible to live a normal life. I try to avoid any kind of force; I cannot have a regular job, and even the commitment of a relationship is difficult, actually impossible. I try to avoid any pressure from the outside world. I suffer from a permanent fear of the police, and due to the same I avoid any visit to doctors. In fact I live in a world dominated by these memories, and they have practically ruined my life. For all this, for all what has happened to me I blame my state, my country. But, I also feel the responsibility lies with those who 'just followed their instructions' and who forgot or refused to show humanity. Yes, I do often think about committing suicide. There is nothing left to live for.'

This visit by the police meant for Heinz, a mentally vulnerable man, the famous straw on the camel's back. It opened the gate, and from then on he could no longer cope.

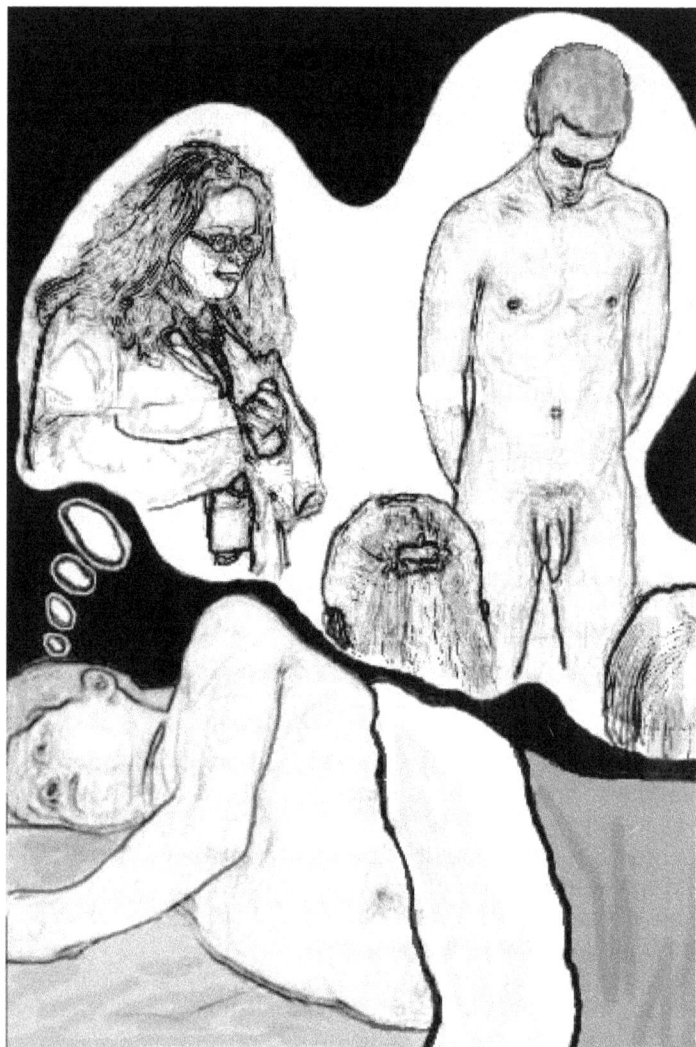

Medical Rape

Easy Prey

For obvious reasons most young people do not want to go to the armed forces or serve in civilian areas as conscientious objectors. In times of peace they find all this unfair and discriminating. Therefore they want to be declared 'unable' and be allowed to get on with their own lives and not with something that is imposed on them. But, with that approach they also make themselves extremely dependent on the doctors in the draft offices. After all, the one who obediently strips and does what he is told might have a better chance to leave as a free man than the one who stands up for his right not to be humiliated.

And, one more thing that could speak against trying to resist to much: even if a person in fact *would* manage to refuse here in this place, the whole matter would still be repeated in the barracks later, and there, as a soldier, a renewed refusal would be seen as refusing to obey orders, a serious military offence that would be dealt with in a much harsher way. So, the prospects are not good. Why not just let them do what they want? Yes, that's what many say and do. But, many will also for years to come regret such a 'decision' or - probably better expressed - subservient approach to the matter. Haunted by their memories, they will deplore they didn't stand up for themselves and defend their dignity.

Unfortunately, after it's all done it's too late to change. You cannot pretend it never happened. Now it is about coming to terms with it and moving on. However, for many people that is not as easy as it may sound, and it doesn't make it easier for the individual that the problem is 'invisible' in society, a no-go-area, something charged with shame. Even if a whole nation in reality knows what has been going on and what is still going on, the same whole nation just tries to ignore it. Victims and perpetrators, they all have an interest in keeping it 'secret'. After all, nobody would openly admit that also he once stood there with pulled back foreskin and spread buttocks. No, nobody would be happy to declare such in the public arena and risk being ridiculed as a consequence. And no such honourable professional would want the world to know what she really is up to at work either. So why not just unite in effort and keep a lid on it all?

No, if the whole issue is ever talked about, it is more likely that the victim will try and describe it all as pretty harmless: 'oh, with *me* it was nothing special really.' Much here reminds me of what we know about victims of other sorts of abuse. Also with them, suppression, either consciously or sub-consciously, is the rule rather than the exception. At most any cost they will try and hide the pain at the bottom of a very deep sea and prevent it with all means ever again to pop up to the surface. If it ever would, it would be too painful. Yes, for most people difficult traumas are better kept as well hidden 'secrets' (or so they seem to think) - secrets shared only with the abusers.

In 1976 I got to know a student, twenty-two years of age and shortly before discharged from the armed forces. Now it comes what makes me feel chills down the spine as I read your story. This young man had the same problems as the ones you describe. He was unable to engage in proper natural physical love. One evening he asked me fairly aggressively: all right, when will you start criticise me? What will you accuse me of? I said nothing; I just took him into my arms, and then he started to cry as a child. How long he cried I don't know. I only remember that he felt asleep in my arms.'

Anette G.

Whether or not a human being is able to recover from difficult experiences is of course not only dependent on good therapy but also on his/her personality. This personality will of course also play a role in what will in the first place constitute a debilitating trauma for that specific individual, and, not least, it will to an extent decide how he or she will be affected of it. Something that might not be too difficult for one person to cope with can have extremely serious consequences for another. For some people certain events can easily be forgotten, but when it comes to others the same experiences can end up haunting its victim day in and day out for the rest of his/her life.

Of course, there are numerous variations as to how we as human beings cope with life. But one thing is important: very often painful memories can stay with the victim hidden in the

Medical Rape

sub-consciousness for years-on-end. We might think they are gone; we might thing 'it was nothing'; we might think we got away. But, all of a sudden they are back, popping up to the surface. A special situation, whatever it can have been, has caused them to re-appear into our consciousness. That is how it often is with memories of sexual abuse, and forced strip medicals belong to that.

I have noticed that quite a few of the men I have talked to have experienced that the memories of the intrusive examinations have been hidden away for years only to return to haunt their minds because something trivial all of a sudden reminded them of what years ago happened. And, sadly for these individuals, now these memories won't go away again. As a result of all this, these people then find themselves in a very difficult situation, in fact in an outright dilemma: they desperately need to talk, but, as they are who they are and as the whole subject is such a taboo, they would go out of their way to prevent the *musterung* ever to become a subject for discussion.

> 'I ask myself why the genitals can be of such importance. The day I started my civilian conscientious objector service I again had to have it all done. Odd really.'
>
> Marcus Z.

This reluctance ever to talk openly about state approved sexual violence is what for years has secured its survival all around the world. And remember, this is so not only when it comes to abusive military medicals, it goes from there all the way to very serious cases of torture. Forced nakedness plays a part in all this, and, be sure of that, a very important one. It is in fact a 'safe' way of abusing human individuals in the name of the state no matter on what level. It is 'safe' because the abuse leaves no physical marks and because one can be fairly sure the victim will 'happily' help cover up the crime.

For sure, the victim will of course never talk about it; he/she will be too ashamed to do so. For most people it will be easier to talk about having been beaten up, kicked and physically assaulted than to admit having been forced to stand naked in front of others. And, had it been in front of people of the *opposite* sex it would be even worse, much worse. That this is the case anybody in the torture arena would be able to confirm. Therefore women are often used to break the will of resistance of male victims of (military and security service) interrogation - as men can be in reversed cases. Anybody who would like to know more about that could enquire at the US camp in Guantanamo Bay.

Of course, between this American concentration camp and the German draft offices there is only one small however perverted and sick connection - nothing more. Fortunately, one would say. Still, it is so that 'experts', no matter where they are to be found, do exactly know what to do to humiliate and ruin people's lives. These 'experts' are everywhere to be found, also in Germany. In fact, it doesn't seem to matter what the reason is, they will still do the job. They will do it no matter whether it is about getting information out of a terror suspect, as with the Americans, or only to show a young German boy that from now on he has nothing to say - as is the case by the *musterung* examinations.

> 'Once I saw pictures of a *musterung* in a book about the Second World War. A number of naked men stood in front of military doctors and officers. It must have been very difficult for them. My grandfather who fought in both the wars often talked about the "adventures", but he never said anything about being *"mustered"*. Now, as I think back, I find that a bit odd, strange really. But, maybe he was just too ashamed to speak about it. It had probably been easier for him to speak about bombs and grenades, killing and maiming - even massacres. At least so it seems.'
>
> Manfred S.

Difficult to say, but, maybe those who work in these draft offices and by the medical departments within the *Bundeswehr* really *are* unaware of what they do to young people. Maybe they really *are* unaware of the lifelong mental problems they cause with their actions. Maybe they really do not understand that what they do to young innocent boys has quite a lot of resemblance with a very specific era in their country's history.

As I thought about that, I also became conscious about something else, another 'mystery'. In fact, what is it that makes some people think that those very specific 'talents' which were widely to be found in the pre-war and war generations should be nonexistent in the present ones? Why should people living today be so much different? After all, there is no secret that during the time of Mr Hitler there were huge numbers of wo-men who openly admired this man and would do just anything to live up to what he asked of his people. Ilse Koch was not the only one; there were many of her type.

No, it is not so that one gender has a monopoly on what is good and that the other has a monopoly on what is evil. As is the case with some men, also some women would happily take part in mistreatment of other individuals - not only on a physical but probably far more so on a mental level. Here I think the circle is about to close: if a person harbours such perverted wishes why not look for a job where they can be lawfully practised? Why not go for a job where sick dreams can be allowed to be carried out in real life?

No, the German draft offices, the German medical services within the armed forces or the state health services dealing with the conscientious objectors, none of them are small Guantanamo camps. Still, there is only a grade of difference when the talk comes to sexual methods to suppress people and make them into obeying tools in the hand of the power.

Lars G Petersson

Long Term Damage

Sexual abuse can have grave immediate as well as long term consequences for the affected person. What I have come to realise is that symptoms often described in connection with other forms of sexual abuse also are to be found by some of the victims of the intimate examinations. Many of these people describe conditions like: depressions, loss of trust, anxiety, sleep disturbances, night mares, an unbearable hate against anything that can have the slightest to do with the trauma, and, not least, suicidal thoughts.

At this point we really need to ask some very serious questions. For example: How many young people have killed themselves because they couldn't come to terms with the shame? How many have beaten up their partners as a result of built up aggression? And, how many have had their sexuality ruined or have turned into addiction - all of it just because they felt humiliated and abused by their own state and its willing cohorts?

As a matter of fact, I don't know. Of course I cannot present any evidence for what I am suspecting. But, from Denmark, a country with much better conditions in this area, statistic research (conducted by medical people close to the defence forces) clearly tells how damaging military service can be to young people's mental health - this without them ever having been close to a war, and this without them ever having been exposed to humiliating medicals as in Germany..... As member of staff in a specific mental health unit under the Danish ministry of defence (speciality: mental breakdowns of conscripts...) I was close to the people behind this report.

One could say that sexual abuse is a sexual or sexually related act that is being committed against the will of another human being - somebody either mentally or physically inferior to the perpetrator, or somebody dependant on him/her. As a victim a child would always fit into that pattern. As he/she cannot even *be allowed* to 'consent' to any sexually related act, everything coming close must be seen as abuse.

In a child/adult relationship the adult is in charge, and, if it is so desired, he/she can do as he/she pleases. In the case of a young soldier or soldier-to-be this part of crossing boundaries has been taken over by the state. So, when the rulers then by

Medical Rape

proxy - without invitation - invade this young person's privacy the outcome is the same. Just like the case with the child, how can it be anything but sexual abuse? No, just as the child that finds itself in the hands of the paedophile, this young person in the hands of the state has got no chance. None of them can defend themselves.

Yes, that's how things are. And, it doesn't really matter if one is only seven and in the hands of the paedophile or seventeen and in the claws of the state-approved inspectors. Both authorities use their powerful positions to scare their victims into submission and compliance. Both I call abusers.

> 'Before I could start working as a conscientious objector, I had to be examined once more. What I found extremely difficult this time was that another (female) doctor entered the room while I was being examined. They started to chat about their weekend experiences, as I lay there stark naked on the couch. Even as it got even more intimate and more humiliating they just continued chatting as if it was nothing special. That was the worst I have ever experienced.'
>
> Jürgen K.

Normally we picture men as perpetrators of sexual abuse: 'women do not commit such atrocities'. However, that is not correct. In fact, we know that in about every tenth case of child abuse a woman is responsible, and if we only count boys the number will increase even further.

How is it then that there is so little talk about female abuse? Why is this phenomena so little known? Is it because it might be more difficult to discover because it might often take place in care situations, an area where abuse is fairly easy to disguise as a professional act? And/or, is it because the general public have difficulties to realise that sexual abuse has more to do with the abuser's head than his penis, and that 'he' doesn't even need to have one?

No, of course not, a perpetrator needs no erection to sexually violate somebody else. After all, sexual abuse is much more than sheer penetration. He needs not fit the stereotype picture of a perverted old man either. No, he can be a fully 'normal' person, socially well functioning and ordinary in most any areas of life. He can belong to most any social class and profession, and he can also be a '*she*'....

In fact, those who abuse others for their own sexual pleasure they are everywhere to be found and they don't all look alike or wear long grey coats. No, as we all know by now, they can be found among clerics, among teachers and, not to forget, among medical and care staff. Not least they can be found in military establishments, and, if we look back at what we have read this far, right there it might be a bit crowded.

Yes, many there will fit into this picture. Because, if you without invitation and without credible medical reason grab out after other people's genitals then you belong to that category yourself: then you are a sexual predator. There can be no question about the following: regardless if one (as a member of staff in any of these institutions) performs these 'examinations' oneself or if one is only acting as a privacy-intruding spectator, in both cases one makes oneself guilty of sexual harassment of defenceless human beings.

There is no excuse for such behaviour; it is not possible to hide behind orders and instructions. Sexual abuse is a criminal offence. The safeguarding of the individual dignity is not just clearly written into the German Constitution, it is also part of the German soldiering law and, not least, it constitutes the very basic commandment also in the medical code of conduct.

In this connection I would also like to remind people about the fact that there *is* something called 'humanity' and that it would be a good idea to practise it. If for nothing else it is wise because we all risk one day to end up at 'the other side'. Sooner or later most people will end up dependent on other people's good will. The day that happens even the *musterung* doctors and their assistants desperately will hope they will be treated in a compassionate and lenient way. It is easier to ask for it if one has practised the same principle oneself.

Medical Rape

At the 'Shunting Yard'

Again and again those responsible are asked to do something about this question. But, it seems to be of no avail. As usual when it comes to questions which cannot easily be dealt with also this one is being sent back and forth between the institutions; it is being sent round in circles - all in the hope, or so it seems, that the problem (with the complainants) sooner or later will just go away.

And, if there is ever a response to any letter, then it will always be the same empty words which are there to be read. Yes, it is quite remarkable: they all remind me of each other no matter from where they come.... In fact, in order to deal with people like myself they, the public servants, seem to help each other. Responses and explanations - all of them showing no understanding of the real problem - all look the same. It doesn't really matter if they come from those (officially) representing the system, the Ministry of Defence, or from the Parliamentary ombudsman, whose job it is to mind (or so it is being said) the interests of the soldiers.

No, no matter from where the 'answers' come, it will always be the same: the difficult questions will, if they are not completely ignored, just be 'misunderstood' and the reply will have very little to do with what was originally asked. Alternatively, in order to make it look as if everything is absolutely in order, statements will be issued to questions which were never asked - all of it making the answer to appear serious and thoughtful even if it isn't.

I am not really surprised by all that, only a bit disappointed. The people who seem to have no desire to protect others go out of their way to protect themselves, and when it comes to that it seems like there are no restraints as regard to what methods can be used. To be honest, it looks like there is only one intention: to make every nagging, pestilential moaner just go away.

Of course, most letters addressed to the authorities about this matter are not replied to. However, from the few exceptions to that rule I have learned a bit about what they, at least as a group, think about it all and what tactics they use to get their way. And, indeed, this can sometimes be quite interesting. Remember, we are talking about people who either make the laws or who live from interpreting them. We would think that at least these guys would strictly stick to the laws and regulations as they in fact are. After all, we talk about *German* authorities, and we talk about their (for strict adherence to rules and regulations) world famous public servants.

Nevertheless, things like the following can happen: laws and regulations which clearly speak *against* the established view that young people just have to accept whatever they are told to endure are simply not taken into account but swept under the carpet. And, at the same time as that happens, other matters, so called 'principles', repeatedly are being made into *looking* like they were more than just that - home made *'principles'*.

We have already mentioned the strange concept of the 'forensic principle' (and especially how it is interpreted to favour the system). And, we have touched base with the strictly home-made principle of 'gender neutrality' (the 'fact' that a doctor is not a he or she but an 'it') and that the person being examined (if he is a man but not a woman...) therefore has no need to feel embarrassed even if the examiner (and her assistant) are of opposite sex in *real* life.

Did that sound complicated? Did you get confused? In fact, if so, then you (and I) are in very good company. Because, when using these strange home-made philosophical constructions, even the people whose job it is to deal with them are not always in full control of their delicate task. Also they seem to get confused and reveal openly that they in fact haven't got a clue what they really talk about.

In last year's report from the parliamentary ombudsman for military personnel this man writes: 'this neutrality in some cases can go missing. This, however, does not change the underlying fact of medical neutrality.' Let us try to forget that nobody really has questioned any so called 'neutrality'. The complainants have only questioned the right to force upon young men privacy-invading examinations, and *that* has nothing to do with anybody's 'neutrality': it has something to do with privacy, decency and dignity, and that is a completely different matter. Let us also try and forget that the ombudsman

Medical Rape

- by using words which were never used in any complaint - obviously tries to divert the question away from what it was originally about.

Let us instead have a look at what this man is actually saying. What does he actually mean by saying that 'this neutrality can in some cases go missing'? As we have already realised that we are *not* talking about the kind of neutrality needed when writing factual medical certificates, so what *is* it we are talking about? The answer is easy to give: it is about 'neutrality' in the meaning that the woman doctor here in this situation is not to be seen as a *female* individual in front of whom a naked seventeen-year-old adolescent male needs to feel (naturally) embarrassed. She is to be seen as a 'human neuter'..., and in the presence of a 'thing' one needs not feel shame.

I have tried to look this phenomena up in the literature, but neither can I find any mentioning of such an odd being in the medical literature nor can I in the complete works of Charles Darwin (though I admit I haven't read it all). No, what seems to exist in the German world of bureaucracy seems to be non-existent in real life of humanity: there they only talk about males and females. Yes, there can be some confusion in single cases, but when it comes to human beings there is generally speaking nothing called 'it'. And, after all, what is important here is not what somebody thinks she is, 'neutral' or not, but how she is perceived by the one who has to strip in front of her.

Before ending this bizarre deliberation, shouldn't we also establish the following: no man would ever be allowed to pronounce himself as 'gender neutral' and thereafter walk freely in and out of female-only saunas.

No matter what we think about this strange creation, what this man, the parliamentary ombudsman, actually is saying is that this 'neutrality *can* go missing....'. And, that's interesting. Not that it actually *can* go missing. Of course it can, because it was never there, but, that this man actually *says* that, that's in itself quite extraordinary.

In fact, what would actually happen if what he says *can* happen actually happens? What would be the consequence of that? Yes, what would happen if a doctor 'suddenly' was to lose her 'gender neutrality'? What is it that 'it' then in fact has lost? Has 'it' all of a sudden become a 'she'? And, if so, who would find out? Who would establish that this transferral actually has happened, and who would report it? And, if they ever were to be reached by this incredibly sad news, what would the Ministry of Defence do about it?

Shouldn't we be straight and honest? Of course, the chance that the ministry would ever get a case to 'investigate' is fairly slim, in fact non-existent. Therefore, the only lesson I can draw out of this story is the following: the ombudsman acknowledges that doctors 'in some cases' abuse their power in the way stated in this book, but he also lets us know that it doesn't change anything about anything - nothing needs to be undertaken as a consequence of that conclusion. Because, if he really meant action was needed, why hasn't he already set all wheels in motion?

'Yes, at the *musterung* a man will be examined by a team of women who themselves never have had to go through the same. That I feel extremely humiliating and unfair. Also that other people have been given the right to decide over my life I find wrong.

'The female doctor at my last *musterung* obviously didn't like me. She must have seen me as a malingerer. When it came to my physical ability to serve she had already made up her mind before she even had had a look at my penis. My breathing problems, asthma? No, she wasn't interested in that....'

Winfried A.

Medical Rape

Sorry, We Have No Opinion

Let us now go back to the public bodies in general and look at how they deal with matters like this one. First, sorry to have to say so, if what you have read this far hasn't given reason for much optimism, what will come won't change that for the better. Let me express myself frankly: I *am* shaken by the indifferent approach these public servants have shown to this serious matter. In the course of the campaign against this abuse, in which this book plays a part, I have had quite a few negative experiences. Basically, these people cannot be bothered.

Only at *one* single moment I have sensed a tiny bit of humanity being shown. After having declared that his minister would not deal with this matter and that I would have to go to the (...guess) Ministry of Defense, he, the public servant, finished his letter with sincerely wishing me good luck with the book.

Yes, that was an exception, though a nice one. All the rest of what these people ever write is passing-the-buck-nonsense. 'Sorry, we cannot answer those questions; it is not within our area of responsibility.' 'We will forward your questions, and you will hear from somebody in due course.' This way critical questions continue to go in circles - with the hope from their side of course that the complainant sooner rather than later simply will give up.

Also, it is striking that it is always the same questions which are avoided, which are left unanswered or which are 'misunderstood'. Most prominent of them are questions regarding (reversed) inequality between man and women, medical relevance of the examinations and, not least, the persistent breech of Article 1 of the Constitution.

For all institutions involved it seems as if certain choices of words must have been carefully prepared somewhere centrally for them all to use. They are at all time, no matter from whom they are sent, almost always identical. Indeed a remarkable set of co-incidences.... Yes, it is all the time the same echoed, meaningless manifestations and the same useless 'explanations' I hear. All in all, it is like if they just refuse to understand the problem, as if they are from another world - and, maybe they are.

155

Worst of it all, however, even worse than being ignored, is when I have to read nonsensical constructions as the one stating that the doctors and assistants have been through 'sensitivity training' and therefore there should be no need to worry.... Of course, I am sure they haven't, but, even if they had, what ridiculous nonsense.... It only shows these people haven't got a clue what they talk about, or, should I rather say, they won't give a damn. Because, if they were really honest, wouldn't it be more 'sensible' simply to spare young people from being victims of this ill-treatment?

Contrary to earlier time in history today mainly women are putting young men into embarrassing positions. And, also on a bureaucratic level, mainly women decide on behalf of them how much they have to endure - all of this, in its own odd way, backed up by the concept of 'equal rights' at the work place. Yes, they decide what is right for these young males, and overall they seem not to care that much for those at the receiving end of the game.

In one letter that has come into my hands a female official at the ombudsman office writes that 'it is true that also young men can feel embarrasment'. She continues to say that it is 'correct and normal for them to feel so'. But, thereafter she also states that 'the institution of the ombudsman has in recent years only received one single complaint from a *directly* affected person' and that the examples in the complainant's letter 'are old'. With that last comment she then dismisses the complaint.

I find this tragic. After all, it is well known that victims of abuse in most cases (and especially when we talk about children and young people) are only able (if ever) to deal with their trauma years after it actually happened. People working for such institutions *must* know that. Therefore, such an approach to such a serious complaint is nothing but shocking.

Yes, this indifference shown by those who *could* make a difference is indeed sad. Because, had this woman had the slightest interest in finding out more, there would have been nothing to stop her. She could have gone everywhere to find it, even to the Parliament itself. Yes, why not to the German Parliament's *own* website for young people (www.mitmischen.de)? There, on 17th July 2009, 'Alexis' writes that '*mus-*

terung and induction examinations are absolutely humiliating. Twice I was examined exclusively by female doctors; one respectively two female secretaries just watched.'

Would the director need more to convince herself of the seriousness of this matter, why not also have a look at the study *'Violence against Men'* commissioned in 2004 by the Ministry for Family Affairs, Elderly and Young People? A look there would no doubt be useful for her. In chapter 5.2 in this study it is said: 'during the *musterung* I had to present my genitals for a woman and thereafter bend forward. ... It was absolutely humiliating, but I had to do it.' The study's comment on that is that the '*musterung* can be seen as an invasion into the private area that can be everything from unpleasant to humiliating.'

Of course, most of all this negligence in action does not surprise me. After all, this is the way authorities deal with many difficult issues. However, that *one specific* organization has chosen to join the choir *does* indeed surprise me. Yes, it is indeed astonishing that precisely the *Deutschen Bundeswehrverbandes* declares that this is not within their area of responsibility. Yes, that *is* truly remarkable. After all, this independent organization's fundamental responsibility is precisely that: to protect the interests of its 200 000 *members* (among them conscripted men and enlisted soldiers of all grades). Nevertheless, for this particular question, the one plaguing so many of its members, this organisation has absolutely no opinion.... but refers to others within the forces.... And we know who they are....

Dissent Within the Ranks

Fortunately for future generations it seems like the strict dis-
cipline enforced on people working for the system has not
succeeded completely in its attempt to shut out every dissi-
dent opinion. Problems are popping up here and there. Yes, it
is clear that not all involved want the status quo to continue. I
am, for example, aware of one female doctor who within a
week quit her job at a draft office, as it was clear to her that
she didn't want to dehumanize people as part of her work.
Due to heavy criticism from BASTA and associated people a
sharp debate between the institutions has also started. It is
obvious that responsible people are trying to find excuses and
ways out, in case the house of cards finally will cave in.
Indeed interesting is that even within the Ministry of Defense
itself an initiative has been introduced to help deal with the
increasing number of critical questions. The main objective:
try and stop this subject from reaching public attention.

There is no question: everything that *can* be done to protect
the system *will* be done, and, be sure about that, it *is* being
done. Still there are people who dare challenge the system.
For years the German Federal Medical Board has had a
complaint on the table. In this document a complainant describes and criticizes the humiliating examinations. Part of this
document has been leaked to me by a friendly source with
access to such complaints. Thanks to this person I can here
disclose what this *insider* has to tell.

Some of these experiences are indeed remarkable: in one
example it is referred to a young man who is in the process of
having his genitals examined. The female doctor had, as it is
described in the complaint, 'been manipulating so much with
the penis that the young man had got an erection and was
standing like that with a red face right in the middle of the
room'.

Now something quite extraordinary follows: as the examiner
thereafter wanted to examine the testicles, they were gone....
disappeared! Faced with this inexplicable 'mystery' the woman panicked and a male doctor was called into the room to
assist. Fortunately for all involved this man was then able to
explain for his female colleague that when having an erection
it is fully normal that the testicles disappear up into the ingui-

nal canal. Indeed comforting news for an incompetent doctor, but it would probably be very difficult to name a more humiliating and degrading situation in which one could find oneself than the one in which this young man had been placed.

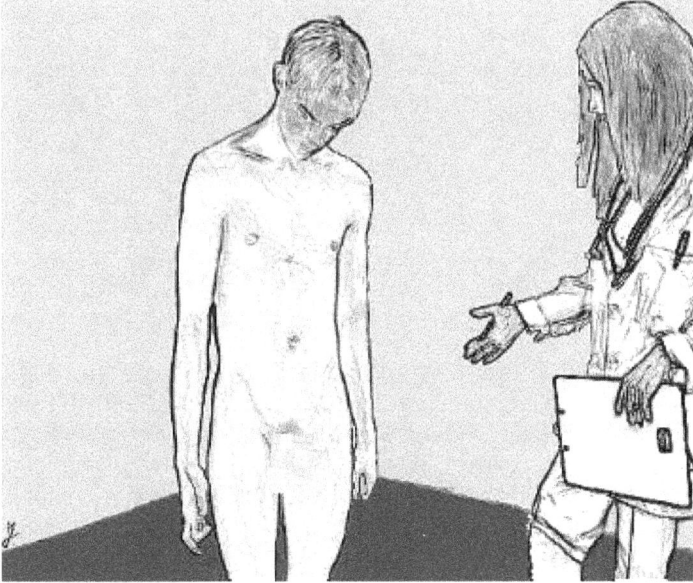

I have heard quite a lot by now, but still, that story shocked me. It was, however, just an example. In another that is also described in this complaint a young man is laying stark naked on a couch in the examination room. He is in full view of everyone present. Again a male colleague is called upon. This time he is asked this question: 'are the genitals here not to small?'

For me it is difficult to imagine a lower standard of 'medical' competence and a more appalling way of behaving oneself. Is it really so that these people believe they can expose young human beings to such sexual abuse with impunity? And, how would a young vulnerable person under such circumstances ever be able to defend himself against such a blatant attack on his human dignity? After all, normally there are no witnesses to speak out on his behalf, and, according to the authorities, there *shouldn't* be any.

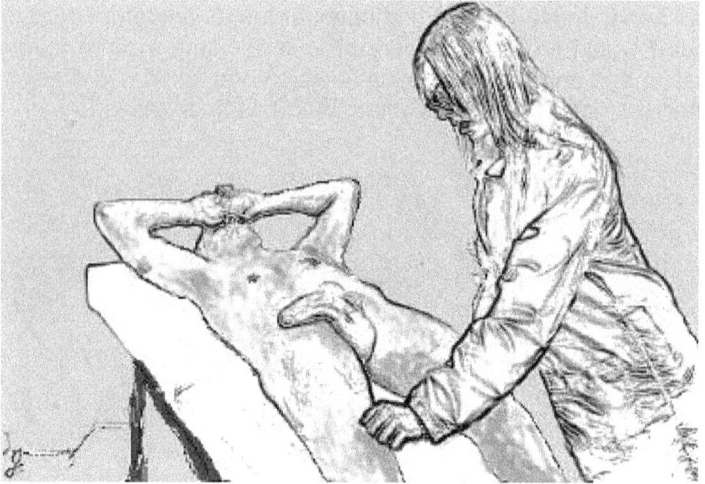

Precisely so: in the rules and regulations for these so called medical examinations (*die Zentrale Dienstvorschrift*) it says clearly that people who are not part of the examination are not allowed to be present. This way the person who is to be examined is automatically excluded from having someone present to protect his interests.

However, for whatever reason, the exclusion seems not to include the female assistants, even if their job, according to the same set of regulations, is strictly limited to entering the medical observations into the files after the doctor's 'dictation'. Note: there is nothing here that indicates they have a part to play in the examination itself. In other medical settings secretaries would compleate their writing work *after* the examination has taken place. Why should it be different here? No, there is absolutely nothing saying that they should be allowed to be present as witnesses.

Medical Rape

Flashbacks

Young people are generally easier to mould and form than those experienced by years gone past. Misused this can have very serious consequences. Child soldiers, for example, are known in many conflicts around the world to be the most violent of all soldiers - all that because of their young age when starting training. Yes, to those just starting out in life it is possible to do what would be extremely difficult if tried with mature adults. This fact is common knowledge and widely used. Anyone who is in power and wants to attack other people knows that. So it was from time immemorial and so it is today.

Precisely, nothing has changed. Young people do not possess the mental maturity to defend themselves against exploitation and therefor they can be sent of to wars and conflicts of which they have no idea what it's all about. Yes, knowing that, can there be any surprise that young people no later than at age 17-18 all around the world are called up to learn the craft of killing?

For military powers it is a great advantage to be able to influence such young people, individuals who haven't really started their life yet. Would the recruitment and/or the conscription start at a much later age (why not at age 35-40?) then it would all look very different. If choosing that path, people in power would face quite another resistance - a completely different challenge. Sure, people who have been given time to develop into independent individuals with their own will, they wont just let themselves be (mal)treated by others in the way as is the case with our youngsters.

Therefore, better start early; therefore, better start in childhood or at least no later than at the end of adolesence - when they are still legally under-age, or at least not long after.

So it is, no matter if we talk about government troops or guerilla fighters in conflict-infested areas in Africa, Latin America or Asia or if we speak about the 'friendly' Bundeswehr in the today peaceful Europe. They all have no problems recruiting. Young people cannot defend themselves. Either they are conscripted or 'attracted' because of poor civilian job opportunities or outright unemployment.

In order to prepare for war it is not only essential to learn aggression and violence in general terms, but, let's face it, also to learn how to rape the enemies' women (this way breaking down their morale). Today it is taboo to say this, but not long ago - as the Nazis still ruled the roost - it wasn't.

As in so many other cases of so called 'defence' also at that time it was not about building up armed forces in order to protect own borders. As we all know, the plan was to attack other countries and to suppress other nations. With help of the self bestowed right to use miitary power at ones own discretion the plan was to start an extermination process where millions of useless, inferior people should be done away with. Only with the help of the armed forces and the conscription law this would have had the slightest chance to work. Only with the help of the army and their drafted soldiers this program of ethnic cleaning would be protected against interference from foreign forces.

Looking at the time of the Nazi rule it is easy to see how young people with help of a conscription law could be made into cohorts for a criminal regime. But the Nazis were no exeptions, only extreme. In many societies all over the world young people continue to risk being exploited and abused in older generations' wars and 'campaigns'.

No, that principle did not die with Hitler. It lives on. Young people continue to be taught aggression and violence by their own states, and, in some places, German speaking countries included, the whole process continues to start with mental abuse of themselves. No, that part of the past has never gone away. It is like if one has never learned the slightest from the horrors of history.

In a modern society of the twenty-first century this is indeed a very serious contempt for the real needs of the growing up generation. All right, many people who have been through this 'school' might claim to be 'mentally undamaged' and might even look as if they were. But, very rarely it is like that. In order to learn how to use violence on command a person has to change his mind-set, or, alternatively, have somebody else to change it for him. And, as we have already seen, there are a long range of methods which will help see that happen. Many of those will qualify as damaging to a person's mental well-being.

Medical Rape

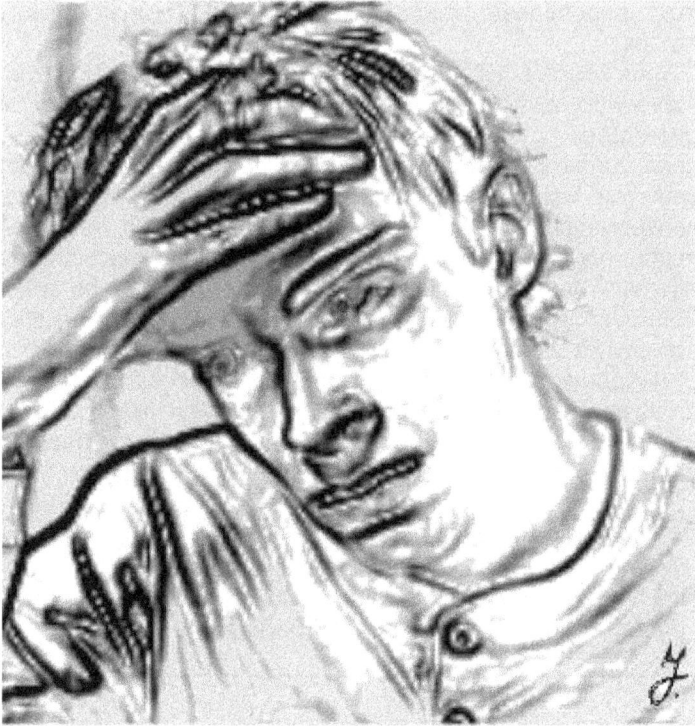

It is not only people with *extremely* brutal experiences in their baggage who might be seen as suffering from what in now acknowledged as the post traumatic stress disorder (PTSD). In fact, what one person could live through without too big a mental scar can change another for ever. For the sensitive and vulnerable, a relatively small trauma can have serious consequences for this person's future well-being and make him or her into a fully qualified sufferer without ever having been anywhere close to an armed conflict or other catast-rophe.

  Not only can I report a number of such cases from a special psychiatric unit for traumatised Danish conscripts in Copen-hagen in which I once worked, but the same I have also found among men who have served in the German armed forces. None of them was ever as a soldier in a foreign country and they were never involved in armed combat. Still they suffered from experiences which had been part of their military training.

Unfortunately, when it comes to some nations, not even those who never made it all the way to the barracks can be guaranteed not to have been damaged. In fact, as we have seen numerous examples of here, also these people can be seen as victims of traumatising experiences with severe consequences for the rest of their lives. Yes, even those who might only have been *mustered* once or twice or trice can be affected. Yes, also among them we meet people who suffer from ever returning horrifying memories. The victims feel they are always there, back in the traumatic situation. The feeling of desperation, helplessness and extreme anger is common for these people. Often even minor things - like a special voice, smell or just anything - can remind about what happened and provoke a flashback into the past.

'To compare it with rape is tempting. The victims cannot defend themselves against the examinations. Still it is all legitimised by the state and obviously accepted by the overall population. Quite extraordinary really.'

Norbert P.

Medical Rape

A Distorted Sexuality

I have touched on the subject before in this book. Now I can no longer avoid trying to explore it a bit deeper. Therefore, let us have a look at the effects this whole matter can have on a young person's future sexuality. Let me be frank: it frightens me to think about how a young person's sexuality due to this kind of humiliation can develop into masochism and what is worse....

Yes, of course, this is another massive taboo, but, we still have to address it. After all, in the context of the complex human nature when it comes to sexuality, this whole matter can very well be the start of a very unfortunate development in a young man's life.

If we like it or not, people who have been exposed to sexual humiliation might, if the preconditions are there, start to feel *aroused* by the very thought of this otherwise *unpleasant* experience. If that is happening, then a sort of sexual perversion has started to take over. If lucky, it stops with that, with a *masochistic* sexuality, a need to feel humiliated in order to reach sexual satisfaction, but, we can never be sure.

Yes, it could get worse. As with so many other things in life also when it comes to this matter there is a range of possible opportunities. One of them would be this one, something that we could allow ourselves to see as a *slightly* worse scenario on the path down a very slippery slope: in his head the person starts to adopt the *dominant* role instead of the passive; he starts to feel satisfied only by the thought of exposing *others* to degrading treatment, or, one step further, he begins to live his dreams in real-life sadomasochistic relationships.

Some might now feel it's all over the top. But, remember, we are all different human beings, and even at this stage (on condition that all participants are volunteers) it can most likely all be accepted as only a variation of an endless variety of individual sexual dispositions. After all, if nobody is hurt or abused, who is to decide what is right and what is wrong?

However, really bad, and now with no question mark attached to it, the problem is if it goes beyond that boundary - if non-volunteers would be exposed to the same. Having said that we are back to where we started: if somebody finds pleasure in humiliating young people in the concept of forced medicals, then he or she belongs here among the other perverted souls.

Yes, there is no question: sadomasochism plays a role in the military examinations. Of course this must be the case if one finds satisfaction in having a job where one can force oneself onto defenceless young people's genitals. But, is that something to be proud of? I thought not. At least I would have thought everything would be done to hide it. In fact, most of the time it is, but, as we are all humans, sometimes people forget, and when that happens we are shown the real nature behind the facade. Believe it or not, the knowledge that some people can find pleasure in sexual domination of others at work has even been used from *official* side when looking for 'suitable' medical staff.... As we have seen before, it has been included as a kind of 'aperitif' in an advert when trying to fill a vacancy at a draft office. As this advertisement is so absolutely extraordinary, here it comes once again:

Advert for Position by the Armed Forces

(This is NOT a perverted joke, author's comment)

Since about a year Ms Dr X works as *musterung* doctor at the *Bundeswehr* draft office in Y-stadt. After ending her medical studies at the University of Essen, she looked for alternative areas of career and discovered the armed forces. The job as *musterung* doctor has turned out to be exactly as she expected it. Now the thirty-three-year-old's work day starts at 7.15 am with the first conscripts.

'Of course it's embarrassing for them when the trousers have to be dropped. And there are so may rumours about these examinations. But, most young men take it all fairly relaxed. I have even experienced that some are happy that it's being done by a female and not a male.'

www.karriere.de/beruf/arbeiten-bei-der-bundeswehr-8315/5 - 67k - **Cached**

That ad is indeed astonishing, but, apart from the fact that it so openly discloses what it's all about, it doesn't really surprise me. After all, in the research for this book I have come across so much that all confirms what the ad implies.

Nevertheless, all of this shows how dangerous and damaging this vicious circle is. On the one hand we have this pleasure in humiliating defenceless young people, and on the other we have all the erect penises representing emerging (involuntary) masochism. Together the two sides represent a perverted sex game played out in cover of health service.

'Due to the memories of my *musterung* I have never attended a medical screening. And, no matter what happens, I never will.'

Konrad B.

Must be Willing to Adapt

When thinking carefully about the whole matter, it is difficult to avoid asking oneself one very important question: isn't it all - not only the intimate part - just extremely out of date?

To be honest, if it really *is* so, that all this exclusively *is* about deciding whether or not somebody is strong and fit enough for service in a twenty-first century army, does it then make sense just to check weight and height, listen to his heart and lungs and 'ask' him to do twenty squats? Wouldn't they then rather have to talk about introducing a modern physical endurance test, at least one on level with what any local gym would be able to perform?

And, seriously, should it be too much to ask if these tests could be performed by somebody who actually knows what he or she is doing? After all, one has every reason to question the qualifications of these examiners. For example, have a look at this ad for a post in Cologne. The requirements are not really to be impressed by.

'Qualification requests: qualified medical practitioner with experience in issuing attests who is able to work in a team, has basic knowledge of modern information technology and who is willing to adopt to the speciality of musterung examinations.'

That means that anybody who has qualified as a doctor and knows how to use a computer is seen as fully competent to decide over life and freedom of other people. He or she will thereafter be given the right to force young men to nakedness and he or she will thereafter be given the power to decide whether they are to be 'acquitted' or alternatively ordered to serve one year of forced labour either in the military or in the civilian area. Yes, it is true, that is all the qualification required for this extremely powerful position.

So what do these people actually need to know? After all, what the advertisement hints at might be sufficient: they might not need to be more qualified. The reason for that could be the following: As everywhere else in society, also within the German armed forces there is a question about supply and demand. Therefore one should not take the question about

Medical Rape

strict 'ability' to serve too seriously: it is more about selecting the number of recruits the *present* political situation actually needs. Right there the line will be drawn for who is able and who is not. The doctor's job will then be to move the bar up and down to match the needs and let enough people (but not too many) pass the requirements. When doing that, it might even be a disadvantage to be too qualified and independent in medical and physiological matters.

How can I say all that? Maybe because if physical and mental ability to serve as a soldier really was that strictly cut in stone, then it would in fact be quite remarkable that the numbers of able-bodied young people always fit so well the numbers needed at any given time.... No, the criterion for being found able will of course be adjusted to the needs of the military and the political situation. The bar will be moved up and down as required. How else could it be that today in the time of the EU there are so many more young men who are considered incapable than at the time of the cold war? After all, in those days, on both sides of the German/German border, the large majority was seen as fully fit for service. And, further back, how could even children during the reign of Mr Hitler be seen as able bodied enough to be sacrificed on the battle field?

In order to show in detail what we talk about, let me present a few figures: in 1990 only 12 % of potential conscripts were deemed unfit for military service in Germany. In 2005 the share had gone up to 40%. A reason for that is easy to find - and it has nothing to do with health and fitness. Of course, the physical standard of young men had not deteriorated that much in only fifteen years. If it really had, it would have been nothing but a national catastrophe. No, in the real world more people were seen as 'unable' because *fewer soldiers were needed*. As a consequence of *that,* and not because of individual health problems, more young people were seen as 'unfit' for service. If it hadn't been so, then it was indeed lucky for Hitler that his generation was in such a fantastic good shape compared to Merkel's....

So, with less and less tension on the political stage more and more young people can have reason to hope they will be lucky to escape the army. On one hand that is of course very good. However, on the other it might have consequences. At least, it will make it easier to realise the increasing power the individual *musterung* doctor will have over the individual young person. Basically, she now has his immediate future totally in her hand. She decides whether he passes the 'test' and is 'rewarded' with a year service or whether he 'fails' and can go home and look after himself. The decision is in her hands.

In that situation this woman is not a person to challenge. Therefore quite a few young people would be tempted to say: 'better let her do what she wants with me. After all, then she might show mercy and free me from service.' Sexual humiliation as alternative to conscripted war service? A questionable choice - especially when (if the gambit does not work) you could have both....

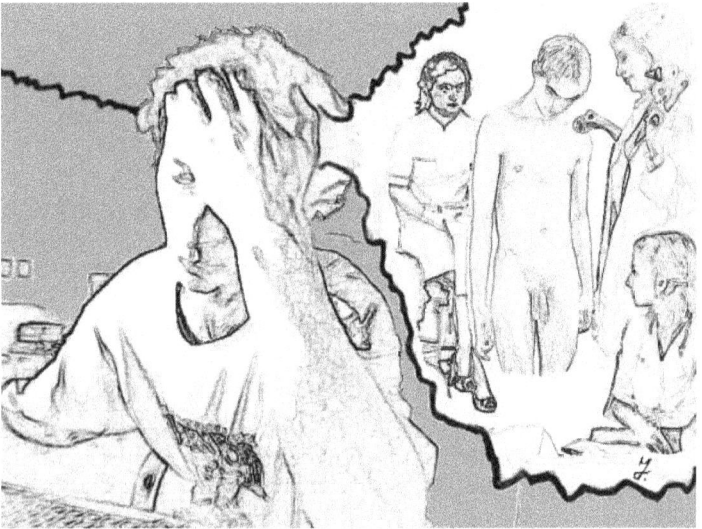

Medical Rape

A Massive Strip Show

Violation of young people's dignity at the conscription offices, by the military and by the civilian authorities responsible for conscientious objectors' non-armed replacement-service is a very serious problem in this part of the world. After all, it is not an issue about some single cases of personal abuse. It takes place on a massive scale, and it is with full approval of the state; in fact, it is all done in the name of the state.

Every year at least 400 000 German young men are obliged to submit themselves to these examinations, and for most of them, as we have seen, one time is not enough: it can all go on and on. On top of these *musterung* examinations (examinations to decide young people's ability to serve in the armed forces) we can every year add hundreds of thousands of similar examinations both at the beginning as well as at the end of service. Note, this goes both for those who serve by the armed forces themselves and for those who have opted for replacement service as conscientious objectors. And, if anybody thought so, it doesn't even stop there: we still have to count all similar abusive examinations conducted on *enlisted* soldiers in order to reach the final number.

To be honest, when it comes to the professionals I am at a loss. I have no idea how many times these young (and even older) men have to strip in order to make the authorities and their doctors happy. However, one thing is certain when it comes to them: as professional soldiers they are just expected to accept whatever they are told. To refuse would be close to impossible. In the end, that would be disobedience, a serious military offence.

By faithfully holding on to and accepting perverted medical examinations, the German people and its representatives are drawing shame upon themselves. This shame must be even bigger when we think about the fact that most of these young people - while having had much of their constitutional rights of protection automatically taken away from them - never even have been given the chance to vote in an election. Precisely so, due to their young age nobody has ever asked them what they want: it has all been decided for them. Against such a group of defenceless human beings - who on top of this find

themselves in a very vulnerable phase of their personal development - the state and its authorities obviously find they can
do as they please.

It is important to remember: such a system of state-sanctio-
ned abuse can only survive into modern time thanks to the
mutual silence of both victims and perpetrators. Also, it can
only survive because most involved people know that should
it ever come to a show down, then there will always be a way
out. There will always be an exit for perpetrators at this level.

Not that I need or want to give any advice here, but, yes,
there are numerous options to follow. Some are better than
others, so why not make it easy and just apply the same
simple defence strategy as has been used so many times
before when officials have gotten into trouble? Why not just
declare that 'I have only acted strictly in compliance with rules
and regulations in force' and/or 'I only followed orders'? Both
those explanations almost always do the trick; together they
are close to fool proof.

To be honest, if also this story one day will end with a swarm
of such pitiful escapes, then it will not be for the first time that
will happen. History, not least the German, is full of similar
examples. Therefore, shouldn't we - as we are now well into
the twenty-first century - rather seek to ban such statements
and shameful excuses to the dusty archives of history?
Shouldn't we rather start making people responsible for what
they do to others? I think that's a good idea. I think it is about
time.

Medical Rape

What Had Happened to Tim?

In the spring 2009 the young German Tim K. went on a killing spree, leaving fifteen people and in the end also himself dead. In the wake of the massacre the whole nation tried to find a reason for the tragedy. How could this happen? That was the question being asked all over the nation. It is true, it wasn't the first time a young person went berserk and killed people, so what has gone so fundamentally wrong?

At the time of his early death Tim K. was seventeen. According to a psychologist, he had lived his last years in a lonesome fantasy world centred around his computer: violent *ego-shooter* games had taken over his life. But, there was more to the picture: on his computer he also collected pictures of bondage scenarios. The parts different people played here were always the same: men were dominated by women. They were chained and exposed to pain.

Something very deep inside this young man must have plagued him terribly. But Tim never talked with anybody about his innermost thoughts. Was there really nobody out there in whom he could have had such confidence? Was there really nobody out there with whom he could have shared his despair? Possibly not. Was shame and embarrassment part of the reason for that? Possibly so. In fact, it seems like Tim had developed further and further into a kind of masochistic submission, and it is equally likely that he wasn't very proud of that. The only thing that obviously made his whole situation mentally tolerable was that he knew one day he would get his 'revenge'. Only so he could live, and, apparently, only so he could die. The possibility that Tim K. on purpose went out to kill *women* is reality; it is very much possible in this case of mass murder. The question that needs to be asked is: 'why?'

Tim K. was not the only young man with such thoughts. He is now dead, but, for sure, there are a number of them out there. In an insecure world, a world in which more and more youngsters - in the absence of good male role-models - withdraw to their computer games, they might be counted in thousands if we are not to talk about tens of thousands or more. I don't know. I have no idea how many they might be. Nobody knows. Equally, I don't know whether or not Tim K. had already been to a *KWEA*, to a German military conscription office. I don't know whether or not he already had been humiliated there in real life. I don't know if he had already been paraded naked in front of the women inspectors and their willing helpers. However, one thing, I do know: the combination of state-prescribed abuse and the sensitive mental world of young men can be a very dangerous mix.

Until recently Mrs Ursula von der Leyen was German minister for family affairs. In this position it is not only about caring for the well-being of families. Mrs von der Leyen was occupied with something 'bigger' as well, namely the preservation of the people itself, regeneration and reproduction - in fact the very existence of the nation. As the young generation also was part of her area of responsibility, it was obvious that also she and her ministry in the process of researching this book had to be asked for their opinion regarding this subject. However, no surprise, neither the minister nor her officials showed any interest in the problems around the *musterung*. I was simply told that this subject (the medical examination of men's genitals) is to be dealt with by the Ministry of Defence.... I cannot understand that, to be honest. To me it sounds a bit absurd. Maybe the ministry and Mrs von der Leyen's successor, Kristina Köhler, would rethink that in the future? At least I hope they will.

In the meantime I am asking myself a question: could it in fact be that I have completely misunderstood something? After all, it was so that the ex-minister's political success-rate while in office especially was tied up closely with the birth-rates of the country. That was much of the reason for why it at the end came to look fairly dim for her. In 2008, one of the years in which van der Leyen ruled over the German families, less children were born than at any time before. Germany was actually to be found at the very end in a European study comparing different countries' fertility rates.

Many women, especially graduates, in fact don't want to have any children at all, and, it seems as if Mrs von der Leyen and her ministry has not been very successful in doing anything about that. All right, she has privately done more than her bit, but, she has failed to get her sisters on board. Now the great responsibility for the fertility of the nation rests on

Medical Rape

Ms Köhler's shoulders, and we will see what she can do. A solution to this problem must be found, or so they say.

Wasn't it so that the survival of a country has something to do with defence of its borders (jobs for the boys) AND with giving birth to children (apart from needed help to get started, wo-men's business)? As already mentioned before in this book: Germany is neither threatened by the Danes nor the Dutch. In fact, there are no other threats either, and, as a consequence of that, modern defence-strategists have long ago left behind the idea of a ready-for-battle-type Hitler/Napoleon mass-army. Precisely so, the idea of such a machine is hopelessly outda-ted; nobody needs that anymore.

But, not to have enough children, that really means some-thing. So, will the Ministry of Family Affairs soon make up its mind regarding how this very serious problem is going to be addressed? Thinking about it myself, maybe it might not be such a bad idea to follow in the footsteps of Dictator Ceau-sescu? After all, both clinics and staff are already there. Only the doctors would need a few minutes re-training.

***

Epilogue (From the Internet)

'Hallo Friends. I have also been mustered, but it wasn't in the old East Germany; it was somewhere even worse - in the former Soviet Union. The year was 1976 and I was just seventeen. We were around fifteen young men in the group that morning. First we were all told to strip of everything and wait like that until being called. After a while a woman assistant called my name, and I had to follow her - totally naked - along the corridor and up some stairs. There, after first having had my eyes tested, I was called in to a fat, young woman doctor. With her were another two females, probably secretaries.

'The doctor called me to step forward. I was asked to stand with my legs spread and the arms behind my neck. She had a thorough look at me before she took the already fairly stiff penis in her hand and examined the testicles. After that I was asked to turn round and bend forward. While I was standing like that she spread my buttocks a bit more, and in that moment I was totally stiff. Of course she had a good laugh. "Oh, you have a nice big one."

'After that I was ordered to do ten squats and the same number of push-ups before one of the other women came forward and brutally ordered me to jump. As I tried to cover my erect penis with my hands, she screamed at me to keep them behind my neck. I had no other chance than to jump as I was told. My head must have been red from shame. After that I was ordered up on the scales, and my length was measured before I finally was asked all possible questions. It didn't seem to me as if the answers interested her, only my organ.

Ako
13.05.09

Someone calling himself 'Ich2408' commented like this: 'oh, what an exaggeration! You can go on any talk show with that.'

'Hello, no it is not exaggerated what I wrote. There is a difference if one is fifty or just seventeen. In that young age a person is extremely vulnerable. With me it wasn't done, but with a friend of mine following happened: after he had first been through roughly the same as me, he was told to lay on a

Medical Rape

couch and lift his legs high up so that the lady doctor could look at his bottom from behind. Dreadful, isn't it? Maybe that was how it was like at a slave auction in the Middle Ages.'

Ako 14.05.09

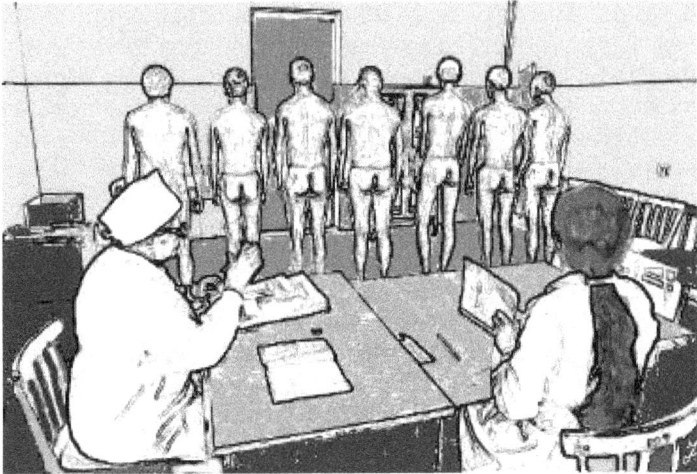

A picture from Russia

Lars G Petersson

Afterword

While writing this story, I constantly had a few lines from the works of the late Danish poet Halfdan Rasmussen in the back of my head. He once wrote it for Amnesty International, and it is about torture.

I am not claiming that also *this book* is about torture. However, it is about degrading treatment, and those two concepts are often mentioned in the same sentence - also in the Universal Declaration of Human Rights, proclaimed and adopted on 10th December 1948 by the General Assembly of the United Nations. There it is written in Article 5 that 'no one shall be subjected to torture or to cruel, inhuman or degrading treatment or punishment'.

Halfdan shared that view, but he also felt that there can be something even worse out there. I know it might be easy for somebody like me to say so (after all, I was never myself put on a rack), but I do understand what this most beloved poet tried to say. Therefore I like to share his words with you in my own very free and utmost humble English version.

It's not the torturer who scares me;
it's not the hate, suffering or pain.
Neither is it the rifle they might point at me,
nor the ghastly shadows down the lane.
No, it's nothing of that that hurts me,
what it is is the blind indifference,
Yes, all these ordinary people who do not give a damn.

www.ingramcontent.com/pod-product-compliance
Lightning Source LLC
Chambersburg PA
CBHW031203270326
41931CB00006B/390